GUIDE TO TRACK AND

FIELD INJURIES

by Arnd Kruger

& Helmut Oberdieck

First English language edition published in 1978
by Tafnews Press,
Book Division of Track & Field News,
Box 296, Los Altos, CA 94022, USA

Originally published as *Kleiner Ratgeber fur
Leichtathletik-Verletzungen,* Verlag Bartels
& Wernitz KG, Berlin, West Germany, 1975.

Standard Book Number 0-911520-85-6

Printed in the United States of America

Cover Design by *Ann Harris*
Production assistants: *David Gleason, Grace Light, Debbie Sims*

TABLE OF CONTENTS

INTRODUCTION

Very often athletes are stymied in their development by various kinds of injuries. Track and field, which leads the human body to the border of physical ability, has a huge number of athletes who have suffered from one injury or another, causing an untimely end to a promising career. Many of these injuries need not have occurred in the first place, had adequate preventative measures been taken; others would have taken far less time to heal if the right measures had been taken promptly; and many others would have been cured much faster and more completely if the medical treatment had been accompanied by the proper exercises.

Yet there are still many track meets where no experienced physician or trainer is present. Even more often, neither one is present at workouts. This means the responsibility for the immediate action after the injury occurs rests with the coach and with the athlete him (her)self. And what takes place in the first 15 minutes after the injury decides to a large extent the duration of the injury and the length of the cure.

Therefore, this book addresses those on the scene immediately after the injury. We do not want to interfere with the duties of the physician, nor do we plan to tell the physiotherapist what to do.

Instead, we have teamed up as former athletes and as coach and physiotherapist, gathered our experiences, and discussed them with a number of physicians, other physiotherapists, coaches and athletes the world over. So you will find not only the German experience of Helmut Oberdieck, three times the Olympic Games Masseur for the German women's track team, but also some American advice through Arnd Kruger's experience at UCLA's smoothly-functioning training complex.

The majority of cures, however, are down-to-earth, time-tested advice which is sufficiently available in literature and in practice, but is so spread out and so little systematized that we brought it together and organized it into a system. And since this book has been on the German market since 1975, it can be said—the system works.

There is no sentence reoccurring in the book as often as the one: "the workouts do not need to be interrupted but. . ."; and this can be considered the basic philosophy of the book. An injury only disturbs a part of your physical conditioning. If you want to keep it up you have to continue to workout with those parts which are still in use in such a way that you keep in shape.

We have therefore divided the book into three parts:
(1) We give a step-by-step description of the common track and field injuries and tell what to do, in which order and by whom.
(2) We have split the workouts after the injury into three phases: a compensatory workout, a curing workout and a preventative workout, for the respective events.
(3) We give an overview of how the various forms of physiotherapy effect the body to make sure that certain workouts and certain regenerative measures are well coordinated and do not interfere with one another.

Let us have a look at the three parts. The advice in (1) is no collection of hints for self-medication, as we think that the peculiarity of every individual case should be carefully observed by the expert physician and physiotherapist. Yet very often this expert is not available so that the coach and the athlete themselves have to take certain measures. It is here that our advice comes in, telling who should take responsibility if a very general diagnosis and a very general prescription of therapy is recommended.

Under (2) we have divided the chapter into the separate events of track and field. We have long considered including additional ones for juniors and seniors and for decathlon and pentathlon. But injuries are very seldom due to a particular age. The youthful organism is particularly injury-prone in joints and ligaments as they are not yet very firm. The injuries there, however, can be treated like the same injury in someone of a different age. The same is true for the seniors, although there is a greater than normal frequency of injuries due to the inelasticity of joints and ligaments, and they may take a little 'longer to heal as the natural growth process has slowed down; the injuries and their treatment, however, remain basically the same. There are few if any typical injuries for the decathlon. The decathlete may get a pulled muscle in the long jump, but then there is very little difference between this pull and the one suffered by a long jumper—they can be regarded as one. Typical injuries due to the senso-motor change from one decathlon event to the other do not occur, for all practical purposes.

In the case of all track and field events we have differentiated between *traumatic* and *technique-related* injuries and problems. This differentiation seemed necessary as the rehabilitation exercises depend to a large degree on whether the injury is automatically connected with the proper performance of the event (i.e., by simply doing it beyond the physical limitation of the athlete at that particular time)—or whether the athlete made a typical movement error which was responsible for the injury. In the long jump, e.g., a knee injury can be regarded as *traumatic* as the stress on the knee, even when properly jumping, is so great that an injury may result and render the athlete incapacitated for some time afterward. If the heel is bruised in the long jump, however, it is only *technique-related* as it is the consequence of an incorrect technique. In the workouts following, some rehabilitative training jumps may be taken up much earlier, since in proper jumping the heel does not touch the ground in a way that it gets bruised in the first place.

Of course we could not list all injuries in this subchapter, but with some common sense all injuries will be found somewhere along the line; e.g., the pull of a long jumper in the run-up is basically the same as the pull of a sprinter, so it is only listed once (under sprinting). Athletes in some events may find themselves underrepresented. This is not because we thought that their events cause less injuries, but that in their cases there are fewer injuries which can be identified as either traumatic or technique-related. If they are spread over the possible spectrum of injuries, they are very difficult to list, and should be looked up under the most similar kind of injury and adapted with some common sense.

We have designated those exercises as *compensatory* which should be used until the injury has healed to the extent that the actual trouble spot can be used, too. If one function for a certain performance cannot be done, others have to be stressed to maintain conditioning.

In the "curing workouts," the injured parts are actually used in isometric or isokinetic training . Isokinetic training has proved to be advantageous for rehabilitation as it adapts the weight applied on the muscle to the strength of the muscle under a certain angle and thus makes sure that the injury does not reoccur by abrupt dynamic motion. In contrast to isometric training it has the advantage of using the muscles at all angles and thus avoiding the disadvantages of a prolonged isometric training at certain angles, i.e., an unbalanced motion curve of the muscle. Isokinetic training requires either an "intelligent" machine to adapt itself to the strength of a muscle at a certain angle or it requires that one does the exercises against the resistance of one's own body—which suffices for rehabilitative purposes.

In the preventative workouts, the exercises are continued up to the full training load and possibly even beyond. Unfortunately the preventative training is very often the last link in a chain meant to prevent the reoccurrence of an injury rather than the first occurrence. It is possible, however, to have a thorough check-up to find out whether certain muscles or tendons are unproportionally weak, and thus, one might start with the preventative workouts at the beginning rather than at the end. For the purpose of systematization, we have left them at the end.

In the third and last chapter of the book we repeat a theme that we have already dealt with elsewhere. Very often the coach does not know the effects which certain physiotherapeutic measures have on the body; similarly, the physiotherapist is not aware of the workout the athlete did before nor of its effects. We have tried to systematize these to help them understand each other better, in order to avoid an over- or under-loading of the athlete. The athlete's body responds to every stimulus, so the coach should try to control as many of these as possible to assure a maximal performance and reduce the possibility of an overload.

Finally, a few words of thanks should be extended. The mutual cooperation of the two authors dates back to 1963, when Helmut Oberdieck cured a trauma injury of Arnd Kruger's in nine days, helping the latter to win a championship, for which he had given up all hope. The win helped him to get a track scholarship to UCLA where the able trainers Alvin "Ducky" Drake and Larry Carter used completely different treatment techniques with considerable success—and were patient enough to answer the tiring questions of an eager German sophomore. In 1968 we participated in the Mexico Olympics where we again had the chance to watch physiotherapists from around the world, and Helmut Oberdieck received a lot of hints from Marvin Roberson of Provo, Utah.

In 1971, when Arnd Kruger completed his Ph.D. and became the first editor of the West German coaching bi-monthly LEISTUNGSSPORT, the question of physiotherapy was dealt with from the very beginning, and Helmut Oberdieck was one of the first to report his experiences there. Out of this cooperation came the idea to systematize the knowledge and give it to the athletes. The book turned out to be a best-seller in Germany, where nothing comparable was on the market. In the spring of 1977 Arnd Kruger was back in the U.S. and his old friend Fred Wilt became interested in the material, since the basic assumption is international: too many athletes are thrown back in their progress when injuries are not properly treated from the beginning. Arnd Kruger translated the book, and David Gleason of *Track & Field News* was good enough to do the proof-reading on the sometimes very German-sounding English.

DEFINITIONS

ABC-Plaster—Compound formed of equal parts of aconite, belladonna, and chloroform, used to reduce inflammation.

Comminuted—Multiple pieces, as with fractures of the bone.

Ethyl Chloride—A compound which, when topically applied, quickly freezes the injured area temporarily.

Fango Packing—Mud from thermal springs which is applied to joints to reduce swelling and pain.

Heparin—Substance derived from the liver which helps to minimize blood clotting.

Ichthyol Packing—A fine, oil-based bitumen or tar, which is applied to joints to reduce swelling.

Meniscus—Cartilagenous tissue which serves to cushion, lubricate, and protect the area around joints.

Periosteum—Membraneous covering of bones.

Periostitis—Inflammation of the Periosteum.

Salt Packing—Towel is soaked in water as hot as tolerable; salt is put on one side of the heated towel, and wrapped around painful spot; second, dry towel is wrapped around to conserve heat; renewed when inner towel gets cold or dry.

Synovial Joints—Refers to virtually all major joints of the body; any joint with a hinge or ball-and-socket configuration; inner lining contains a lubricant, or **synovial fluid.**

TYPES OF INJURIES AND
HOW TO TREAT THEM

MUSCLE CRAMP

A more or less long lasting, painful, involuntary muscular contraction, which does not disappear with normal muscular activity. Its most common form is the calf muscle cramp.

The most common causes for muscle cramp: deficiencies in ionization (lack of salt due to excessive perspiration); lack of calcium; undissolved waste-products of fatigue in the muscles; narrowing of the capillaries due to insufficient training; psychological disturbance of the nervous system (due to stress situation); tie up (ligature) of the blood system (too-tightly tied shoes, too-tightly fitting clothing, too-tight taping, bandages etc.); sudden, violent exterior pressure (being kicked or elbowed, etc.); too-long-lasting static muscular contraction (e.g., in isometric contractions, in "set" position of the crouch start, in everyday habits such as car driving); bad circulation in an area of former injuries.

First action: remove any pressure from the affected muscles. In the case of a leg cramp, for instance, lie down on the spot sideways on the non-involved side; leave the leg in the position that is least painful; have yourself carried to a suitable place (if there is no stretcher available, hop on the non-involved leg with the aid of two helpers).

Entitled to assist immediately: anybody.

Most suitable to assist immediately: trainer.

Immediate help: relax; improve circulation in the afflicted area; improve metabolism by resting; open up anything that might constrict circulation; make the body and the affected area warmer (sweat suit; blankets; wet warm compress; take salt tablets; after this, try to stretch your own muscle against resistance.

If this succeeds: cramp disappears. Continue exercises by easy use of the involved muscle for a minimum of five minutes (e.g., jogging on soft surface).

If this does not succeed: continue immediate help measures and try again within the next 15 minutes.

If you do not succeed then, it is no longer a cramp but a more serious problem. The troubled area and the adjacent joints to be covered by a moist, warm compress in the least painful position to calm the muscle. See a physician as soon as possible.

Common mistakes in immediate assistance: an attempt to stretch the cramped muscle violently without any regard for the pain to the individual; or to try to dissolve the cramp by massage-like hard grips and beatings. This heightens the risk of pulled and torn muscles.

Entitled to further treatment: physician.

Further treatment: according to recommendation of physician. Physiotherapy could involve the following possibilities: *on the day of the injury*—15 minutes hot air (150 F); massage (kneading, loosening, and vibration of the disturbed area and the corresponding movement segment near the spine); drainage of the corresponding lymphatic ducts; warm (body temperature) partial baths; keeping the disturbed area covered; renewed hot salt packings on the disturbed area.

2nd and 3rd day: physiotherapy as on first day.

4th to 9th day: treatment as before but the massages may be harder and more locally applied.

Further recommendations: normalize salt input (check for balanced diet); check everyday habits (e.g., avoid long auto trips to meets); increase aerobic training for improvement of capillarization; weight training for disturbed area to strengthen the muscle; check general condition (decrease stressful situations; a vacation or layoff might be necessary); avoid too tight everyday and athletic clothing.

Frequent mistakes in treatment: with a too hard, too early local massage a reverse reaction can result. Trying to heal and strengthen the muscle too early, whether or not the muscle can yet stand a full load.

PULLS

Pulls are injuries of cells and cell connections caused by tearing within muscles, tendons, ligaments, and cartilage due to excessive, insufficient or improper demand on its elasticity.

Pulls are recognizable as a pointlike, stitching pain at the moment of the injury or during later attempts at movement. A painfree position of the muscle or tendon, etc. is possible. When pressure is applied to the spot the pointlike pain reoccurs; when pressure is decreased the pain decreases.

The most common internal reasons for pulls are: mistakes in coordination (muscles working against each other); neuromuscular disturbances within a muscle; disturbance in the central nervous system (e.g., shock); reduced flexibility of muscles or tendons (e.g., due to cold weather or lack of warm-up); local interference to the normal blood flow; too much of a braking action (e.g., in the high jump at the take-off, or in sprinting); reduced elasticity due to a cramp; insufficient elasticity due to high muscle tone; inflammation of the muscle (myositis); infection (e.g., infected teeth).

The most common external reasons for pulls are: overload by too heavy a weight; excessive centrifugal force in rotational throwing (e.g., hammer); disturbed coordination due to exterior influences (e.g., being pushed suddenly in a race); attempting to dissolve a cramp by force; uneven ground; disrupted coordination due to weather conditions (e.g., strong gusts of wind); slipping; under-demand of the muscle due to less resistance than expected (e.g. a discus that slipped from the hand too early).

MUSCLE PULL

First action: stop any motion of the involved muscle. In the case of a pulled hamstring (biceps femoris muscle), for instance, lie down immediately sideways on the non-injured side; put your leg in the least painful position; get carried to a suitable place; if no stretcher is available, have two helpers assist you; limp on the non-disturbed leg.

Entitled to help immediately: anybody.

Most qualified to give immediate help: trainer.

Immediate help: cold, moist compress should be taped unelastically onto the disturbed area. Ice (if none is available, have it brought from the nearest soft drink stand), coldpack or cold water on the afflicted part of the body (up to 20 minutes). Stop any motion of the muscle by an elastic fixation of the adjacent joints. See a physician as soon as possible, and avoid any load on the muscle.

Common mistakes in immediate assistance: continuation of exercise; massage-like handling of the muscle; heat treatment.

Entitled to give further treatment: physician.

Further treatment: according to recommendation of physician. Physiotherapy could involve the following: *on the day of injury*—ice and cold treatment, moist cold compresses might be renewed (no longer than 20 minutes at a time, if ice is used). Then apply inelastic pressure with a bandage; moist ointments on heparin base for fast closing of the interior wound, softening of scar tissue and fast dissolution of blood clots (haematoma). Avoid movement, go to bed, do not use the affected muscle (it may be fixed by a non-elastic tape).
2nd and 3rd day: leave compress but renew the moist dressing by squeezing on more ointment. Avoid moving the muscle. If it is a muscle involved in walking, have it tightly taped and do not move it.
4th and 5th day: healing exercises for the respective muscle, first without, then with additional weight resistance. When there is no pain, add resistance until the normal training load is reached. As soon as the exercise has reached the normal training weight load, massage of the muscle may begin. Maintain moist compresses at night.
6th to 9th day: local massages, lymph drainage of the

involved region; hot air treatments; hot and cold water treatment; underwater massage (whirlpool treatment).

Further recommendations: increase coordination exercises; check salt intake (calcium and sodium); increase aerobic training for better circulation; weight training to strengthen the muscle; check everyday habits and general condition (reduce stress situations, a vacation or layoff may be necessary); check training and competition site for holes and other hazards.

Frequent mistakes in treatment: too early massage, particularly in the disturbed muscle; starting exercise too early, even if the muscle seems able to stand the full load; little or no exercise of the muscle during treatment. Full ability to use the muscle will be unnecessarily delayed unless you exercise during treatment.

PULLED TENDONS

First action: stop any action of the affected tendon by resting the adjacent joints. In the case of the Achilles tendon, for instance, sit down, put the ankle in the least painful position, and have yourself carried off the field. If no stretcher is available, have two people help you, while you limp off on the unaffected leg.

Entitled to give immediate help: anybody.

Most qualified to give immediate help: trainer.

Immediate help: cool disturbed area with ethyl chloride, ice (get it from the nearest soft drink stand, if necessary), cold water or moist dirt. For improved circulation of the adjacent muscles, cold and hot treatment may be used alternately. Prevent movement of the disturbed tendon by firmly securing the adjacent joints (preferably by taping). See a physician immediately, but avoid using the tendon in the meantime.

Common mistakes in immediate assistance: continuing to use the injured tendon (danger of full rupture); massage-like handling of the injured tendon; unnecessary attempts to use the affected joints; bandages which allow the joints to move, insufficiently limiting the range of motion of the injured tendon.

Entitled to give further treatment: physician.

Further treatment: according to the recommendation of physician. Physiotherapy could mean the following: *on the day of the injury*—renew ice and cold treatment (no longer than 20 minutes at a time when ice is being used). Then apply pressure with a non-elastic bandage and ointment compress to avoid swelling, inflammation and small blood clots in the tendon area. Rest the tendon completely, putting it in an elevated position if possible. Place moist hot salt compresses on the affected region, *excluding the injured tendon,* to improve the elasticity of the adjacent muscles.
2nd and 3rd day: renew moist hot salt compresses on the area; instead of the compress bandage, taping may be used; apply dry heat and cold (hotpack and coldpack) in intervals of 20 minutes each; allow complete rest for the involved area, avoiding usage of the injured tendon.
4th to 8th day: local massage of the area, including lymph drainage; fango packings; hot air, light or infra-red treatment; hot and cold water treatment, possibly underwater massage (whirlpool bath).

Further recommendations: increase coordination exercises; check salt intake (sodium and calcium); increase aerobic training for better circulation; check everyday habits and general condition (reduce stress situations, a layoff may be necessary); check street shoes in the case of Achilles tendon trouble; increase amount of stretching exercises for the affected area; check sites of training and competition for trouble spots; for up to four weeks a tape support of the tendon may be necessary; for four weeks, apply heat treatment and local massage directly before a workout or competition and cold (ice) treatment directly thereafter.

Frequent mistakes in treatment: too early massage of the tendon itself; stretching the tendon within the first ten days; attempting to train too early, even if the injured tendon can stand the full load, without adhesive tape support.

PULLED LIGAMENTS

First action: try gently to continue the function of the joint; walk gently to the nearest first-aid station or trainer.

Entitled to help immediately: anybody.

Most qualified to give immediate help: trainer or first-aid.

Immediate help: cool disturbed area by ethyl chloride, ice (get it from the nearest soft drink stand if necessary), cold water or wet dirt. In case of ice treatment it should not be applied for more than 20 minutes; tape the affected joint in such a way that the normal movement of the joint is possible, but not permitting any side movement outside the main range of motion. See physician.

Common mistakes in immediate assistance: unnecessary attempts to move the joint in all possible directions (increases the pull); complete fixation of the joint (the blood clusters will block necessary movements for your particular event and thus prolong the time before workouts can begin again); heat treatment on joint (the blood cluster will enlarge and block the whole joint); no (or loose fitting) bandage or tape (pull may become larger); taping too tightly (decreased circulation will produce other risks, such as cramps, and functional motion may be blocked, thus prolonging recovery time).

Entitled to give further treatment: physician.

Further treatment: according to recommendations of physician. Physiotherapy could involve the following: *on the day of the injury:* cold treatment, renewed wet-cold compresses; then tight fitting cushioned tape, which allows the range of motion that is needed for your particular event; alcohol and heparin or other ointments to reduce swelling, possible inflammations and clotting; moist hot salt packings on the affected body region (excluding the joint) to improve circulation and eliminate blood clots. Renew heparin and other ointments that will help reduce swelling in the joint and adjacent areas.

2nd and 3rd day: continue as on first day but use mild warm treatment (hot water bottle) instead of cold.

4th to 9th day: local massage of the affected area, including lymph drainage; fango packings on the region; hot and cold water treatment; underwater massage; renew heparin packings; leave on properly fitting tape; regularly renew alcohol ointment bandages.

Common mistakes in treatment: stretching exercises for the joint within the first ten days; testing too early whether the joint is fully usable without taping.

Further recommendations: increase coordination exercises; check salt intake (iodine metabolism); increase capillarization by more aerobic training; check everyday habits (shoes and heels in the case of Achilles tendon); check everyday habits (you have have to lay off for a while to reduce stress situations); avoid stretching and flexibility exercises of the injured area; special weight training for the muscles used in functional movement of the joint.

Frequent mistakes in treatment: massaging the tendon too early; stretching exercises for the tendon within the first three weeks; attempting to train too early even if the tendon seems to be able to stand the full workload.

If an operation is necessary, the duration of treatment will be different, as recommended by the physician.

BEGINNING LIGAMENT RUPTURE

This is felt as a stitching pointlike pain. No painless position of the joint is possible. When pressure is applied to the ligaments the pain increases and continues for quite some time, even when the pressure is stopped.

First action: aid gently in the function of the joints; try to walk (even if an ankle ligament) gently to the nearest first aid station or trainer.

Most qualified to give immediate help: trainer.

Immediate help: cool disturbed area with ethyl chloride,

ice, cold water or moist dirt for up to 20 minutes; put a tight-fitting tape around the joint, permitting movement that is typical for your event but does not allow any additional (side) movement. See physician immediately.

Common mistakes in immediate assistance: unnecessary attempts to move the joint in all possible directions (increases rupture); complete fixation of the joint (clotting prevents functional movements and will therefore prolong the time before regular workouts can be resumed); heat treatment (the joint will swell and the clots will jam the whole joint); no bandage or a loose-fitting tape (will interfere with blood circulation and prolong absorption of clots; further, tight taping does not leave the joint functionally mobile, lengthening the time before workouts can be resumed.

Entitled to give further treatment: physician.

Further treatment: according to the physician. The physician may recommend an operation. If physiotherapy only is recommended the following is advisable: *on the day of the injury:* renew ice and cold treatment, wet cold compresses; then employ a cushioned tape bandage with alcohol ointments in the cushion, taped in such a way that the typical movements of the joints are allowed; hot, wet salt packings on the adjacent muscles to increase circulation for better absorption of blood clots; use heparin ointment regularly on the joint and the adjacent region.
2nd to 9th day: same as on the first day, but instead of cold treatment, use mild warmth (hot water or bottle or heating pad) on the joint.
10th to 21st day: local massage of the adjacent muscles, including lymph drainage; fango packings; hot and cold water treatment on the joint; underwater massage (whirlpool); renew heparin ointments; leave taping on; renew alcohol packings for 14 days, and stop the heparin after 14 days, switching to ichthyol packings.

Further recommendations: increase coordination exercises; check salt intake (sodium and calcium); increase aerobic training for improved circulation; check everyday habits and general condition (most beginning ruptures are worsened by poor general condition); avoid stretching and flexibility exercises for the joint for at least another month; special weight training for the muscles that are responsible for the proper functional movement and stabilization of the joint.

Frequent mistakes in treatment: stretching exercises for the injured joint within the first nine days; attempting to train too early even if the joint seems able to stand the normal workload without taped support.

If an operation is necessary at the joint (or draining of the fluid within the joint) the start of the physiotherapy and rehabilitation program must be postponed according to the recommendation of the physician.

RUPTURES

The rupture is a complete separation of tissue of muscle, tendon or ligament, caused by mechanical under- or over-demand on its elasticity. It is connected with severe internal bleeding, causing blood clots, which may puff up the skin over the respective area. In the case of muscle ruptures, after the clots are gone there may even be a little dent in the muscle. It is always connected with a reduction in strength and resistance to maximal weight loading.

RUPTURED MUSCLES

The rupture of several muscle fibers is felt like a severe blow. Even in the least painful position of the muscle a hammering, tearing, pressing pain is felt. The muscle has a reduced tone. At its surface a dent may be felt; if pressure is applied at the injured spot the pain immediately increases. These ruptures are generally caused by incorrectly-treated pulls and beginning ruptures (see muscle pull and partial rupture).

First action: stop any movement of the injured part; lie down where you are so that the injured muscle will no longer be used. Have yourself carried on a stretcher; if this is not available have two people support you when being carried to an appropriate spot.

Entitled to help immediately: anybody.

Most qualified to give immediate help: trainer.

Immediate help: put the ruptured parts of the muscle closely together and tighten them with an inelastic tape. Cool the injured area with ice, cold water or ethyl chloride until you see a physician. If ice is applied it should not be used for more than 20 minutes at a time. Elevate injured region. See physician as soon as possible (emergency room of a hospital) and avoid any motion of the ruptured muscle.

Common mistakes in immediate treatment: massagelike handling of the ruptured muscle; attempting to move the injured muscle (in case of leg injury, lie down); seeing the physician (hospital) too late (danger of severe interior bleeding); putting the muscles together too late and the tape too late (the wider the muscles are apart when they start to rebuild, the longer it takes before workouts can be resumed).

Entitled to give further treatment: physician.

Further treatment: an operation may be necessary. Further treatment according to recommendation of physician. If he recommends only physiotherapy the following is advisable: *on the day of the injury:* renew cold packs and moist cold ointments; do not move muscle. Go to bed, or at least stop any motion of the injured region.
2nd to 9th day: (or even longer according to recommendation of physician and depth of rupture): no motion of the injured muscle, if it is a leg muscle, a cast or bed-rest may be necessary.
10th to 20th day: change inelastic taping to moist ointment (heparin) to dissolve the remainder of blood clots and to soften the newly forming tissue; start exercises for the muscle, when these are possible, against a resistance which is close to the normal workout weight; full body massage (excluding the injured region at first!) may be started.
21st to 28th day: local massage including lymph drainage; fango packings; hot air; hot and cold water; under water massages (whirlpool).

PARTIAL RUPTURES

This is a partial separation of cells in muscles, tendons and ligaments which is caused by mechanical under- or over-demand on the muscle's or tendon's elasticity. The pain is felt at the moment of rupture like a severe blow to the whole area, and the injured area remains painful regardless of its position. If pressure is applied to the injured spot the pain increases. The internal and external reasons for the injury are the same as those mentioned under pulls. In fact, incorrectly treated pulls can cause ruptures.

TREATING MUSCLE RUPTURES

First action: Stop movement of the muscle, e.g., in the case of a thigh muscle rupture, lie down on the non-injured side, put the injured leg in the least painful position, and have yourself carried away to a suitable site (if no stretcher is available, have two people help you).

Entitled to help immediately: anybody.

Most qualified to give immediate help: trainer.

Immediate help: Cold and moist compress, which is taped firmly to the disturbed area. Ice (if none is available, have it brought from the nearest soft drink stand), cold pack or cold water on the disturbed area. If ice treatment is applied, it should be limited to 20 minutes at a time. Stop any motion of the injured muscle by inelastic fixation of the joints which the injured muscle normally moves. See physician as soon as possible, avoiding movement of the muscle on the way.

Common mistakes in immediate assistance: attempting to move the injured muscle; massaging or similar handling of the injured muscle; heat treatment.

Entitled to give further treatment: physician.

Further treatment: according to recommendation of physician. If he recommends physiotherapy only, the following is advisable: *on the day of the injury:* ice and cold treatment; moist, cold compresses; if ice is used, it should not be applied for longer than 20 minutes; then inelastic pressure-applying bandages, moist heparin ointment for fast closing of the interior wound, softening of scar tissue and fast dissolution of blood clots (haematoma). Avoid motion, go to bed, or at least stop using the injured muscle.

2nd to 5th day: leave compress but keep it constantly moist by squeezing in more ointments; elevate the injured area, if possible; avoid motion of the injured muscle; stay in bed, if possible.

6th to 9th day: exercises first without then with weights, increasing up to the normal training load, but avoiding additional pain in the muscle. If the normal training load is reached, local massage on the injured muscle may be taken up. Renew moist ointment packagings at night.

9th to 14th day: local massages including lymph drainage; fango packings; hot air; hot and cold water treatment; underwater massage (whirlpool).

Further recommendations: increase coordination exercises; check salt intake (sodium and calcium); increase aerobic training for improved circulation and capillarization; special weight training for the injured muscle to build it up to a higher degree than before; check everyday habits and general condition; increase flexibility training; check training and competition sites for uneven spots; renew training, using a supportive tape at first.

Frequent mistakes in treatment: massaging the injured muscle too early; exercising too early even if the muscle seems to be able to take a full load; exercising too late or not at all, which of course will prolong the time needed for regaining complete use of the muscle.

BEGINNING TENDON RUPTURE

This is felt as a stitching, pointlike pain. No painless position of the tendon is possible. When pressure is applied on the tendon the pain intensifies and continues for quite some time even when the pressure is stopped.

First action: stop moving the tendon by no further action of the adjacent joints; e.g., in the case of an Achilles tendon beginning rupture: sit down, put the foot in the least painful position, have yourself carried away on a stretcher or, if this is not available, by two helpers. Do not use injured foot.

Entitled to help immediately: anybody.

Most qualified to give immediate help: trainer.

Immediate help: Cool disturbed area with ethyl chloride, ice (if none is available have it brought from the nearest soft drink stand), cold water or moist dirt up to 20 minutes. For improved circulation of the adjacent muscles cold and hot treatment may be used in turn. Cease any movement of the injured tendon by taping the joints which are supposed to be moved by this tendon; see a physician as soon as possible; avoid using the injured tendon.

Common mistakes in immediate assistance: continuation of use of the injured tendon (beginning rupture may turn into complete rupture!); massage or similar handling of the injured tendon; unnecessary attempts to move the adjacent joints; taping which still permits movement of the tendon.

Entitled to give further treatment: physician.

Further treatment: according to recommendation of the physician. The physician may recommend an operation. If physiotherapy only is recommended the following possibility is advisable: *on the day of the injury:* renew ice and cold treatment (no longer than 20 minutes at a time when ice is used); inelastic pressure-applying bandage with an ointment compress to avoid swelling, inflammation and clotting in the tendon area. Completely rest the tendon, putting it in an elevated position if possible; moist hot salt compresses in the area around the tendon (but not over the tendon itself) to improve the elasticity of the adjacent muscles and reduce the deterioration of the muscle tone.
2nd to 9th day: renew moist hot salt compresses on the area; instead of inelastic cushioned taping, now use a tight

fitting taping; hot packs and ice packs, 20 minutes each, as many repetitions as possible; complete rest of the injured region; avoid using the injured tendon.

10th to 21st day: local massage of the area, including lymph drainage; fango packings; hot air, light or ultra red light treatment; hot and cold water treatment on the area; underwater massages (whirlpool).

Further recommendations: increase coordination exercises; check salt intake (sodium and calcium); increase aerobic training for better circulation; check everyday habits and general condition (reduce stress situations, a layoff may be necessary); check street shoes in case of Achilles tendon trouble (they may not provide correct balance); more stretching and flexibility exercises for the injured area; check training and competition sites for trouble spots; support the tendon with tape during maximum load training and competition for four weeks; regular massage of the area for four weeks, including heat treatment beforehand and ice treatment immediately after workouts.

Further recommendations: increased coordination exercises; check salt intake (sodium and calcium); increased aerobic training for better circulation and capillarization; special weight training for the injured muscle; check everyday habits; check general condition (you may be overstressed and need a lay-off; include more loosening and stretching in the training program; check workout and competition sites for dangerous spots.

Frequent faults in treatment: massages started too early, particularly of the ruptured muscle; exercising too early even if the muscle seems able to stand the full load; because of too late or insufficient exercises, unnecessary prolonging of time before workouts can be started with full load; taping of the muscle right after injury, either too loosely or kept on for too short a time; discarding too soon the recommended motionless position of the muscle; taking off the uncomfortable moist ointment bandages too early.

RUPTURED TENDON

The rupture of a tendon is felt like a severe blow. The ruptured tendon can no longer be tensed. No painless position is possible. Even in the least painful position there remains a beating, pressing, tearing pain. When pressing at the ruptured site a dent is felt and the pain is worsened.

First action: stop any action of the respective part of the body; lie down where you are in a position that feels the most comfortable and applies the least pressure on the ruptured tendon. Have yourself carried away on a stretcher (if leg tendon) or have two people help you.

Entitled to help immediately: anybody.

Most qualified to give immediate help: ambulance.

Immediate help: None. Get an ambulance to drive you as soon as possible to the emergency room of the nearest hospital.

Common mistakes in the immediate help: attempts to move the joint to which the tendon is attached; any attempts at treatment; delay in getting to the hospital.

Entitled to give further treatment: surgeon.

Most suitable further treatment: operation by surgeon who is experienced with sport injuries of this kind.

Further treatment: operation. After the operation follow the orders of the surgeon.

Frequent mistakes in treatment: delay in having operation.

RUPTURED LIGAMENTS

In the rupture of ligaments some part of the ligament is broken. It is caused by over- or under-demand on the elasticity of this ligament. The pain is felt like a severe blow. The ruptured ligament is only partially fulfilling its function thereafter. No painless position is possible. A tearing aching pain remains which is increased by further kinds of pain (blood and synovial fluid clots).

First action: stop using the joint; if necessary, have yourself taken on a stretcher to the nearest first aid station or physiotherapist.

Entitled to help immediately: anybody.

Most qualified to give immediate help: Red Cross or physiotherapist.

Immediate help: cool disturbed area with ethyl chloride, ice, cold water or moist dirt up to 20 minutes or until arrival of physician; moist cold cushioned taping which leaves the functional path of the joint open but does not permit any side motion. Get to the emergency station of the nearest hospital as soon as possible with the greatest care for the injured ligaments.

Common mistakes in the immediate help: attempting to move the joint; attempting any treatment; late transport to the hospital.

Entitled to give further treatment: surgeon.

Most suited to do further treatment: surgeon who has a considerable amount of experience with athletic injuries in the field of tendons and ligaments.

Further treatment: operation or cast. Further treatment according to recommendation of physician.

Further recommendations: increased coordination exercises; check salt intake (sodium and calcium); increased aerobic training for better circulation; check everyday habits (e.g., heels of normal shoes for uneven wear in the case of Achilles tendon injury); check general condition (reduce stress, you may have to take a lay-off); avoid unnecessary stretching of the injured ligament until it is completely recovered; special weight training for the supporting muscles around the particular joint.

Frequent faults in treatment: attempting to fix the joint with too loose a bandage (elastic instead of inelastic); further use of joint after injury; the rupture may not be properly identified because of the layer of blood clots surrounding it.

RUPTURE OF SYNOVIAL JOINT

Ruptures in synovial joints are caused by an over or under demand on their elasticity. If this takes place the pain is felt in the whole area of the joint. The joint swells up with blood clots and synovial fluid. No painless position of the joint is possible. The injury is generally caused by accidents, e.g., the attempt to lift weights (weight training) one is not yet capable of; unevenness of the ground, slipping, under-demand due to unexpected lack of resistance (discus slipping out of the hand), bad take-offs or landing when jumping.

First action: stop using the respective joints; try to cool it as soon as possible with ethyl chloride, ice, cold water or wet dirt; get to emergency station of hospital as soon as possible.

Entitled to help immediately: anybody.

Most qualified to give immediate help: trainer.

Immediate help: any sort of ice (cold) treatment that can be applied as soon as possible; transport to the nearest hospital.

Common mistakes in the immediate help: attempting to move the joint; heat treatment; delay in getting to a hospital.

Entitled to give further treatment: physician.

Further treatment: an operation may be necessary. Further treatment according to recommendation of physician. If only physiotherapy is recommended the following possibility is advisable, after a 2 week complete rest period:
1st to 3rd week of treatment: local massage of the injured

region including lymph drainage; fango packings; hot and cold water treatment; tight taping to avoid any further rupture, but which leaves the functional path of movement for the athlete's event open; too strenuous exercises for the muscles surrounding the joint, e.g., at first without weight resistance then weight resistance at the normal training load.

Further recommendations: increase coordination exercises; check training and competition sites for uneven spots; increase weight training for the stabilizing muscles of the injured joint.

Frequent mistakes in treatment: attempting to end the inactive period of the joint too early.

INFLAMMATION OF:

An inflammation is a reaction of tissue which appears as redness, increased temperature, swelling, pain or disturbed function and which is due to interior or exterior chemical, mechanical, climatic, nervous or otherwise unfavorable stimuli.

MUSCLES

An inflammation of muscles is the reaction of muscle tissue, which is shown by locally increased temperature, swelling, pain and reduced function and which is caused by stimuli due to the metabolism and the nerves.

The most common reasons for this disturbance are: overstress, lack of coordination, neuromuscular irregularities, local circulation irregularities, repeated cramps or pulls, lack of flexibility of the muscles and/or tendons, unevenness and/or lack of flexibility of the surface for training and competition; lack of elasticity of the muscle due to elevated muscle tone.

The inflammation of the muscle is felt as a continuous pain in the region of the inflammation. It is connected with a continuous tenseness of the muscle. If the muscle is used, the pain in the area increases. If pressure is applied, the pain increases and stays for a while even if the pressure is taken off.

First action: finish competition or workout.

Entitled to help immediately: anybody.

Most qualified to give immediate help: anybody.

Immediate help: apply moist cold packings to the disturbed area, to be renewed when becoming dry; stop unnecessary use of inflamed muscle; see physician.

Common mistakes in the immediate help: massagelike handling of the inflamed muscle; heat treatment; seeing the physician too late.

Entitled to give further treatment: physician.

Further treatment: according to recommendation of physician. If only physiotherapy is recommended, the following possibility is advisable:
First day: stop using the inflamed region; apply moist cold packings for 90 minutes, renewing them when they get dry; repeat treatment after 4 hours; overnight ichthyol, zinc ointment or clay packings.
2nd and 3rd day: do not interrupt workout, although you may have to reduce the intensity; cold and warm water treatment; lymph drainage; repeat packings overnight; check your daily liquid intake, and increase it by drinking teas or juices to increase the function of the kidneys and add some more vitamins.
4th to 9th days: do not interrupt workouts, although you may have to reduce the intensity; lymph drainage and massage; cold and warm water treatment; renew packings overnight, continue the additional tea and juices.

Further recommendations: normalize salt intake; check for balanced diet and adequate minerals and vitamins; check everyday habits (e.g., avoid long drives); have a thorough medical check-up for additional infection and inflammation (e.g., your teeth).

Frequent mistakes in treatment: local massage; heat treatment.

TENDONS AND TENDON SHEATH (TENDOSYNOVITIS)

Inflamed tendons and tendon sheaths are the reaction of the tissue to negative stimuli, which are caused by mechanical or nervous influences, the metabolism, or foreign particles in the body. The inflammation manifests itself as locally increased temperature, swelling, pain and reduced function.

The most common reasons for this disturbance are: lack of coordination; neuromuscular irregularities; local circulation irregularities; lack of flexibility of muscles and/or tendons; repeated attempts to overcome a resistance the body is not yet ready for; repeated cramps or pulls; unevenness and inelasticity of the surface for training and/or competition; lack of elasticity of the attached muscle due to increased muscle tone; inflammation of the attached muscle; infection and other inflammation (e.g., bad teeth).

The inflammation is felt as pain which is connected with the slightest motion of the tendon and which is very locally restricted to the tendon. Pressure increases the pain for a certain time. The inflammation is not felt right away as a sharp pain; it gradually increases, at first appearing only in between running (e.g., in interval training); when the performance is continued the pain increases.

First action: complete workout: if the pain is still there at the next workout, see a physician.

Entitled to help immediately: anybody.

Most qualified to give immediate help: anybody.

Immediate help: moist cold packings on the respective region; when they dry out renew them; fix the tendon, including the joint which is moved by it, in the position that is the least painful; see physician.

Common mistakes in the immediate help: massagelike handling of the tendon and its surroundings; heat treatment; seeing the physician too late.

Entitled to give further treatment: physician.

Further treatment: according to recommendation of physician. If only physiotherapy is recommended the following possibility is advisable:

1st to 9th day of treatment: cold and warm water treatment; lymph drainage; massage of the respective segments; possibly underwater massage (whirlpool); check liquid and mineral intake, and increase it with tea and fruit juices, to increase the amount of water secreted and the vitamin intake.

Further recommendation: increased coordination exercises; increased aerobic training for better circulation; check sites of workouts and competition for uneven ground; regular whole body massages; have a full medical check-up for additional infections and inflammations (e.g., teeth); check everyday habits (e.g., your shoes if tendons in legs were troubled).

Frequent mistakes in treatment: renewing intensive training before pain disappears; too early local massages; heat treatment.

BURSAE

Inflammed bursae are reactions of the bursa of the tendons, caused by negative mechanical stimuli or by particles foreign to the body. The inflammation manifests itself as redness, locally increased temperature, pain, and reduced function.

The most common reasons for this disturbance are: local circulation irregularities; lack of flexibility of the adjacent joint; inflammation of the adjacent joint; lack of elasticity of the respective muscles due to increased muscle tone; infections and other inflammation; bruises; frequent pressure in the area of the bursa.

The inflammation is felt as pain in the case of any movement of the tendon or joint; the pain is locally restricted to the area of the bursa; when touching the bursa with some pressure it can be felt as being somewhat enlarged, hard and inelastic; the pain will linger on after the pressure is removed.

The inflammation is not felt as a sudden pain, but initially can be felt during the intervals when the tendons are not being used. If the reasons for the inflammation continue the pain will be felt more and more during and after each workout.

First action: continue competition or workout to its end. Observe the kind of pain. If the pain does not go away but is felt even stronger in the next two workouts, see a physician.

Entitled to help immediately: anybody.

Most qualified to give immediate help: anybody.

Immediate help: moist-cold packings on the respective area; when they dry out renew them; put the injured tendon, including the joint, in the least painful position; see physician.

Common mistakes in the immediate help: massagelike handling at the bursa, the tendon or the joint; heat treatment; seeing the physician too late.

Entitled to give further treatment: physician.

Further treatment: according to recommendation of the physician. The physician will normally recommend about a nine-day rest. If physiotherapy is recommended the following possibility is advisable:
1st to 9th day of treatment: cold and hot water application; lymph drainage; massage of the respective segments; possibly underwater massage (whirlpool); clay packings; exercises for improved cure; check liquid and mineral intake, increase it with tea (to increase liquid flow) or juices (to improve healing process by liquid + vitamins).

Further recommendations: increased aerobic training for improved circulation; check sites of workouts and competition for uneven ground; regular whole body massage in turn with massage of the joints; have a thorough medical check-up for possible infections; check everyday habits (e.g., alcohol, nicotine, coffee or drug consumption may have to be reduced).

Frequent mistakes in treatment: pain killing drugs or injections; intensive workouts before the pain is really gone.

THE BONE MEMBRANE (PERIOSTITIS)

The inflamed periosteum is a reaction of the skin around the bone to negative stimuli, which may be due to mechanical reasons, foreign particles in the body, the metabolism or the nerves. The inflammation appears as locally increased temperature, swelling, pain and reduced function.

The most common reasons for this disturbance are: local circulation irregularities; lack of flexibility of the adjacent tendons or muscles; inflammation of the adjacent joints; lack of muscle elasticity due to increased muscle tone; faulty coordination; uneven ground or insufficient elasticity of the ground where the training or competition is being performed; inflammation of the connective tissue next to the periosteum; inflammation of the nerves serving the respective area; infections; orthopedic abnormalities (e.g., flat feet, legs of uneven length).

The inflammation is felt as a pain when the respective muscle is used. The pain is felt the most at the beginning and end of the tendon where it is attached to the bone or at the joint. The pain radiates into the whole adjacent area; when pressure is applied to the respective spot the periosteum feels rough and hard and an increased pain continues after the pressure is no longer applied; the inflammation is not felt as a sudden pain, but can be felt especially at the beginning in the intervals when the tendons are not being used. If the reasons for the disturbance continue, the stitching pain will get worse and worse after each workout.

First action: continue competition or workout to its end; observe the kind of pain. If the pain does not go away but is felt even stronger in the next two workouts, see a physician.

Entitled to help immediately: anybody.

Most qualified to give immediate help: anybody.

Immediate help: hot salt water packings; hot salt water

baths; fango packings; ichthyol, iodine ointment or heparin ointment dressing.

Most common mistakes in the immediate help: cold treatment; massagelike handling of the respective area.

Entitled to give further treatment: physician.

Further treatment: according to recommendation of physician. If only physiotherapy is recommended, the following possibility is advisable:
1st to 9th day of pain: renew hot salt water packings; hot salt water baths; fango packings; ichthyol dressing; heparin dressing; iodine dressing; lymph drainage.

Further recommendations: check volume of training—it may be more than can be handled at the moment; have skeletal system checked (some support may be necessary in the shoes); check coordination; increase stretching exercises; regular full-body massage alternating with lymph drainage and local massage; check for infections; check everyday habits (control alcohol, coffee, nicotine and drug consumption).

Frequent mistakes in treatment: pain killing drugs or injections; cold treatment.

THE JOINT

The inflammation of the joint is the reaction of the joint and its components to negative stimuli, which may be due to mechanical errors, foreign particles, the metabolism or the nerves. The inflammation appears as locally increased temperature, swelling, pain, redness and reduced function.

The most common reasons for this disturbance are: local circulation irregularities; frequent mechanical over- or under-usage; faulty coordination; lack of elasticity of the respective muscles due to increased muscle tone; unevenness or inelasticity of the ground; infections; orthopedic abnormalities.

The inflammation can be felt as a pain when the joint is moved; the pain radiates into the adjacent regions; when the area is pressed it feels rough, swollen, and tense; after the pressure is no longer applied, the increased pain lingers on; the inflammation is not felt as a sudden pain but can be felt (especially at first) in the intervals between workouts. If the reasons for the disturbance continue, the stitching pain will get worse and worse after each workout.

First action: continue competition or workout to its end; observe the kind of pain. If the pain does not go away, but is felt even stronger in the next two workouts, see a physician.

Entitled to help immediately: anybody.

Most qualified to give immediate help: anybody.

Immediate help: ichthyol ointments; heparin ointments.

Most common mistakes in the immediate help: massagelike handling of the region of the joint; cold or heat treatment.

Entitled to give further treatment: physician.

Further treatment: according to recommendation of physician; if only physiotherapy is recommended, the following possibility is advisable: *1st to 9th day of pain (maximally 3 weeks):* lymph drainage; local massage; hot and cold water treatment; herbal baths (e.g., tincture of arnica); icththyol or heparin ointments.

Further recommendations: increased aerobic training for better circulation; increased coordination exercises; check workout and competition sites and implements; regular full body massage including lymph drainage and massage; have a check-up for infections; orthopedic check-up (foot support may be necessary); check everyday habits, control alcohol, coffee, nicotine and drug consumption.

Frequent mistakes in treatment: pain killing drugs and injections; manipulation at the joint.

CONNECTIVE TISSUE

Inflammation of connective tissue is a reaction of the

tissue (particularly of the skin) to negative stimuli, caused by mechanical reasons, particles foreign to the body, the metabolism, or the nerves. The inflammation appears as locally increased temperature, swelling, redness and disturbed function.

The most common reasons for this disturbance are: local circulation irregularities; repeated mechanical over- or under-usage of the tendons or joints; faulty coordination; uneven or inelastic ground; infection of the local lymph system; major infections elsewhere; orthopedic irregularities; open infection of the same area; bruises or repeated pressure; ligatures.

The inflammation can be felt at first as a slight continuous pain in the inflamed area; the pain radiates into the adjacent region; the spot itself feels doughy, puffy and tight and is frequently covered by a shining layer of skin; when pressure is applied the pain increases and continues for some time after the pressure is gone; the inflammation does not hurt with a sudden pain, but is felt at first in the intervals between workouts.

First action: continue workout or training to its end; observe the kind of pain; if it does not go away or gets worse, see physician.

Entitled to help immediately: anybody.

Most qualified to give help: anybody.

Immediate help: moist cold compresses on the inflamed area; repeat when getting dry; see physician.

Most common mistakes in the immediate help: massagelike handling of the respective area; seeing physician too late.

Entitled to give further treatment: physician.

Further treatment: according to recommendation of physician; according to size and intensity of the disturbance, the physician will recommend reduced usage or complete rest for the inflamed region; if in addition physiotherapy is recommended, the following possibility is advisable:

1st day until the inflammation is over: lymph drainage in the corresponding segmental region; arnica ointments at body temperature (renew when getting dry); arnica bath for the respective area; calcium permanganate bath for the area; zinc glue or ichthyol ointments; if possible, elevate the area when at rest.

Further recommendations: increased coordination exercises; increased aerobic training for an improvement of the circulation; check competition and workout sites and implements; check-up for infections elsewhere in the body; check everyday habits, e.g., too tight fitting garments; decrease alcohol, nicotine and drug consumption; have skeletal system checked.

Frequent mistakes in treatment: manipulation of the inflamed area.

THE SCIATIC NERVE

The pain is felt at the sciatic nerve and the surrounding area.

The most common reasons for this disturbance are: exposure to cold (e.g., after sitting on cold floor); stress on the spine (e.g , in weight training); infections elsewhere, particularly in the teeth; disturbed metabolism (e.g., lack of certain vitamins); drug, alcohol or nicotine consumption; reduced circulation; local pressure on the sciatic nerve (e.g., by infected spine); birth defect at the 5th vertebra of the spine; injured discs; frequent stretching and twisting of the spine (e.g., by discus throwing).

The pain follows the sciatic nerve. To check whether it is really the sciatic nerve, lie down somewhere level, and lift up the straightened leg; if it is the sciatic nerve the pain will increase along the entire length of the nerve. If the leg is then bent at the knee, the pain will decrease. If while lying, the straight hurting leg is turned inward, the pain will increase along the entire length of the nerve; if it is then flexed in the knee, the pain will decrease; if while lying, the feet of the straight leg are bent toward the body, the pain will increase along the entire length of the leg. When standing straight and lifting the unaffected leg high from the ground, the pain in the hurting leg will increase; when sneezing or coughing the pain may increase.

The following spots are sensitive to pressure: middle of buttocks; fold between buttock and thigh; middle of the backside of the thigh; in the middle just above the bend of the knee; in the middle just below the bend of the knee; side rim of the Achilles tendon; in the middle of the fibula head.

First action: continue competition to its end; during the workout try to find out by the above test positions whether it is really the sciatic nerve; depending upon the severity of the pain, see physician immediately or later; if you can hardly walk, use crutches; if the pain is so severe that the legs feel numb, be carried on a stretcher to a physician immediately.

Entitled to help immediately: anybody.

Most qualified to give immediate help: anybody.

Immediate help: dry heat (infrared light; electric warming pad; hot-water bottle); rest in position that is the least painful.

Most common mistakes in the immediate help: massagelike handling at the tendon which increases inflammation due to the new mechanical stimulus); attempt to stretch legs or spine by force; insufficient warmth in the lumbar region during workout (e.g., wet shirt, wet sweat suit after workout).

Entitled to give further treatment: physician.

Further treatment: according to recommendation of physician. If in the treatment physiotherapy is recommended, the following possibility is advisable: Full body massage, possibly underwater massage; thermal baths; fango packings on the lumbar region and the other painful areas; local massage; infrared treatment; hot air or hot light treatment; hot water bottle overnight.

Further recommendations: coordination exercises for the lumbar region; avoid cooling the skin particularly in the lumbar region (don't sit on cold rocks or ground, avoid short shirts that slip open when bending forward; medical check-up for further infections in the body; control everyday habits (you may need a lay-off from too much stress); balanced diet (sufficient vitamins); avoid alcohol, nicotine, drugs, etc.; have spine x-rayed for possible congenital defects; weight training for the back muscles.

Frequent faults in treatment: cold treatment; cold-moist-treatment; amateur chiropractic handling of the spine; no x-ray control.

BLISTERS

Blisters are a defect in the upper layers of the skin due to mechanical pressure, rubbing or heat, by which fluid collects under the skin. We differentiate between blisters, burns, blood blisters and open blisters.

The most common reasons for this disturbance are: badly fitting socks, badly fitting shoes, particles in the shoes, socks of artificial fibers, unusual movement of the feet in the shoes (e.g., when running up or downhill), mechanical rubbing in the implement (discus, javelin, weights, etc.), burns caused by too much sun exposure, burns on synthetic track after slipping. The blistering is usually very obvious and feels like a wound. In the blister there is air, lymph fluid or a mixture of lymph fluid and blood, according to the position of the tissue.

First action: (1) *In the case of competition:* continue competition to its end. In the case of long distance running, consider running barefooted; in the case of throwing events put a tight-fitting bandaid (available at first aid tent, from a physiotherapist or any pole vaulter) over the blister. (2) *During a workout:* as soon as the pain is felt, take a break and try to remove the cause of the blistering. In the case of blistering in the shoe: get rid of particle in the shoe, straighten out socks (you may have to take off the socks); if it is at the heel, put toilet paper or leaves in the shoe to raise the heel; consider finishing the workout barefooted; throwers may tape the irritated spot or change over to a different part of the workout.

Entitled to help immediately: anybody.

Most qualified to give immediate help: anybody.

Immediate help: Blister—after the workout (and the shower), cut the blister open with a disinfected (e.g., flame-heated) needle, scissors, or tweezers on one side; press out liquid; lift up the skin and stuff the blister with Vaseline, zinc cream or any other fatty cream. Press the skin gently onto the stuffing, attach band-aid to cover the area. *Burns:* treat according to size; in the case of big ones see physician immediately; cover small ones with special powder or jelly; use special band-aids for burns. *Blood blister:* the treatment is done in accordance with the amount of lymph liquid in the blister. If there is more lymph than blood treat like normal blister. If it contains more blood (and has a dark color) leave the healing process to the body and cover the area to avoid further irritations. *Open blister:* clean the area of the wound with a disinfectant; cut off the remaining loose skin without injuring the sides of the wound; remove any particles from the wound (with disinfected tweezers); apply vaseline or other fatty cream; cover area with a band-aid.

Most common mistakes in the immediate help: disregarding the blister and its cause (it may get worse in the next workout); operating on the blister with a non-disinfected implement.

Further treatment: in the case of complications, a lot of dirt or suspicion of infection (risk of blood poisoning and prolonged healing process) see physician immediately and follow his orders.

Further recommendations: cover areas that are particularly susceptible to blisters with tape during workout or competition; control shoes and socks—cotton socks and well-fitting leather shoes are preferable (it may be necessary to enlarge or cut the leather open where the blisters are forming on the foot); make the skin more resistant with hand cream; partial baths with tanning bark; cover susceptible area with artificial resin spray.

Frequent mistakes in treatment: not seeing a physician if pain continues.

SUNBURN

The sunburn is a disturbance of the upper layer of skin tissue due to too much sun exposure (particularly ultra violet rays), after which the skin gets red and irritated.

The most common reasons for this disturbance are: intensive sun exposure without sufficient clothing and/or sun tan oil; sweat on the skin which increases the power of the sun's exposure and by which the effectiveness of the oil may be decreased or washed off.

First action: go to shady, well-ventilated rooms; open tight-fitting clothes; cover skin to prevent heat loss.

Entitled to help immediately: anybody.

Most qualified to give immediate help: anybody.

Immediate help: put sun tan oil or powder on reddened areas.

Most common mistakes in the immediate help: wetting the reddened area; disregarding the danger of the burn.

Entitled to give further treatment: anybody.

Further treatment: in case of small blisters on the skin treat like other blisters. Otherwise repeat application of sun tan oil; painkilling drugs (it may be necessary to take some light sleeping pills for the first night); cover burns with linen cloth; avoid carbonated drinks; increase the vitamin A and C intake.

Further recommendations: prior to further sun exposure, apply more sun tan oil; cover with sufficient clothes and sun hat; avoid unnecessary sun exposure.

INJURIES CAUSED BY ACCIDENTS

SKIN ABRASIONS AND CHAFING

Destruction of the upper layer of skin or its parts are caused by single or repeated mechanical influences. The most common reasons for this injury are: violent external action (e.g., falling); chafing of skin on too tight-fitting sports wear; chafing of skin on skin (e.g., between the legs or between arm and body). The abrasions are accompanied by the oozing of body fluid (lymph or blood) and a pain which is continuous but restricted to the affected area.

First action: In the case of chafing: before continuing workout, try to get rid of reasons for chafing (e.g., if the heel chafes at the shoes put paper in the shoe to raise heel).

In the case of abrasion: get the materials necessary for immediate help.

Entitled to help immediately: anybody.

Most qualified to give immediate help: qualified first aid personnel (e.g., trainer).

Immediate help: In the case of a moist wound: zinc cream or an absorbent powder should be applied to dry up the wound and help disinfection. *In the case of bleeding wound:* Disinfect the wound with hydrogen peroxide; take out any dirt particles from the wound with disinfected tweezers; cover wound with oil or petroleum jelly (e.g., cod-liver oil); cover wound loosely with sterile gauze or cotton; make sure no new infections may arise.

Most common mistakes in the immediate help: washing out the wound with water; covering the wound with non-disinfected material; disregarding the wound.

Entitled to give further treatment: physician.

Further treatment: according to recommendation of

physician, possibly tetanus shot.

Further recommendations—For chafing: put fatty cream (e.g., deer tallow) on endangered area before exercise; check your athletic gear thoroughly (e.g., use tight-fitting cotton T-shirt to avoid chafing of the nipples). *In the case of abrasions:* check competition and training sites; increase coordination exercises; if abrasions come from a sport in which landing plays a role, increase technique training.

OPEN WOUNDS

Cut or rupture of the skin and the layers of muscle tissue underneath due to a single mechanical stimulus from the outside. The most common reasons for this injury are: falling down on a sharp-edged object; getting spiked; injuries with throwing implements.

The open wound is visible as a cut on the surface of the tissue, from which (after a possible delay due to tissue shock) blood will flow.

First action: In case of slow flowing of (normally dark) blood: Get the implements that are necessary for immediate help. *In the case of a blood flow:* close wound with your fingers and get the necessary materials for immediate help. *In the case of pulsing (light red) blood:* Don't become nervous! Press on the nearest artery in the direction of the heart and tie it up tightly about one hand-width away from the wound. Get the necessary materials for immediate help.

Entitled to help immediately: anybody.

Most qualified to give immediate help: first-aid personnel or trainer.

Immediate help: In the case of slowly flowing blood: protect wound with sterile gauze against dirt and unclean air; if nothing sterile is available a clean cloth has to do. *In the case of flowing blood:* stop blood flow by putting the sides of the wound together and binding it with sterile gauze or cloth. *In the case of pulsing blood:* elevate injured part of body. Try to stop bleeding by constricting the arteries, bringing the wound together and covering it with sterile gauze.

Most common mistakes in the immediate help: washing out the wound; pouring disinfectant into the wound.

Entitled to give further treatment: physician.

Further treatment: according to recommendation of physician (he may put in some stitches, give a tetanus shot, etc.)

Further recommendations: after the healing process is over have the scar tissue softened by massage and ointments.

Frequent mistakes in treatment: lack of control by physicians. See also mistakes in the immediate help.

BRUISES AND CONTUSIONS
A destruction of the upper layer of tissue by mechanical stimuli after which no fluid appears on the surface. The most common reasons for this injury are: getting kicked; accidents with throwing implements; getting hit by hard objects. The injury can be recognized by a swelling and a change of color in the contact area; in the whole contact area there is a stitching pain which will feet temporarily increased when pressure is applied.

First action: as soon as possible the contact area should be cooled with ethyl chloride, ice, cold water or moist dirt for up to 20 minutes; if possible put the contact area in an elevated position.

Entitled to help immediately: anybody.

Most qualified to give immediate help: anybody.

Immediate help: continue cooling; elevate injured area.

Most common mistakes in the immediate help: heat treatment; helper tries to move the injured areas.

Entitled to give further treatment: physician.

Further treatment: according to recommendation of

physician, the bruised area may have to be x-rayed to check for broken bone. If only physiotherapy is recommended the following seems advisable: *day of injury to 3rd day:* moist cold alcohol ointment packing as continuous bandage. Keep it moist by refilling the alcohol in short intervals.

4th to 9th day: moist cold alcohol ointment packing as before; heparin packings; lymph drainage; local.

Further recommendations: cover bruised areas with padding if the possibility of reoccurrence is imminent; work on improved reaction time.

Frequent mistakes in treatment: local massage of the affected area; heat treatment; not having the spot x-rayed; disregarding bruises because of other injuries connected with it, e.g., abrasions.

SPRAINS
They can be felt on occurrence or the first movement thereafter as a pointlike pain in the capsule. There is no completely painless position. The sprain of the capsule of a joint is always connected with leakage of fluid in the joint area.

First action: try gently to continue the function of the injured joint; try to get to the nearest physiotherapist or first aid-station.

Entitled to help immediately: anybody.

Most qualified to give immediate help: first-aid or physiotherapist.

Immediate help: cool injured area with ethyl chloride, ice, cold water or moist dirt up to 20 minutes with ice, preferably until you see a physician. Apply moist cold cushioning bandages to fix the joint in a functional position; get to the emergency station of the nearest hospital without delay and with considerable care for the joint.

Common mistakes in the immediate help: attempting to move joint in all possible directions; prolonged time before you go to the hospital.

Further treatment: according to recommendations of physicians. He will normally recommend a fixation of the joint for up to 2 weeks. If afterwards physiotherapy is recommended the following possibility seems advisable:

1st to 3rd week of treatment: local massage of the injured area including lymph drainage; fango packings; cold and hot water treatment on the injured region; taping of the joint that allows for functional motion; exercises to help the healing process—at first without resistance, then (if no pain is felt) increased resistance until the normal workout load is reached.

Further recommendations: increased coordination exercises; check-up of the sites of training and competitions; increased weight training for the muscles that move and stabilize the injured joint.

Frequent faults in treatment: attempt to end the fixed position of the joint too early.

BRAIN CONCUSSION
Functional disturbance of the brain is caused by exterior stimuli; which normally leave no negative effects. The disturbance is connected with numbness or a loss of consciousness and is generally caused by accidents such as getting hit, falling, etc. Other parts of the body may be involved. The disturbance may also be connected with: circulatory collapse, dizziness; decreased blood pressure; the urge to vomit directly after the accident; complete lack of muscle tone; contracted, later dialated pupils which react to light; trembling; clouding of the eyes; lapses of memory.

According to the length of the unconsciousness one differentiates between *slight* (0-30 minutes), *middle severe* (several hours), and *severe* (several days) concussion of the brain.

First action: end competition or workout immediately. Lie down on one side (in case of renewed unconsciousness and vomiting), have head slightly raised. In case of external injuries have them covered by the necessary material. Decrease bruise and head pain with ice packings. Send for physician; if unconscious transport to the nearest hospital.

Entitled to help immediately: anybody.

Most qualified to give immediate help: anybody.

Immediate help: check pulse and breathing until physician comes. Check for possible blood in the mouth (danger of choking!); you may have to remove blood from mouth and nose; you may have to apply mouth to mouth resuscitation; treat additional injuries.

Most common mistakes in the immediate help: insufficiently calm approach; no medical check-up, particularly in the case of light concussions.

Entitled to give further treatment: physician.

Further treatment: according to recommendation of physician or hospital; the physician will recommend normally some days of bed rest *even after light concussions.*

Further recommendations: particularly after light concussions you should see a physician for a follow-up check-up when the acute symptoms are over. If after taking up training and competition new symptoms are recognizable, you should go see a physician immediately. Disturbances in the general health very often mean that you have gotten up from complete rest too early. If the symptoms of the concussion occur without the actual accident, check your running and jumping habits, as they together with an inelastic spine may have the same results on your brain as an acute accident. If this is the case you should do additional exercises to strengthen the back muscles and work on flexibility of the spine.

FRACTURES
Broken tissue connections of the bone by one or repeated forceful mechanical actions. The most common reasons for this injury are: unevenness of the ground; accidents with sports gear; fatigue (particularly in the middle of the foot) caused by rhythmic continuous stimuli (e.g., road running); fatigue due to irregularities in nourishment while there is an overburden of work at the same time.

The bone fracture can be felt as: an abnormal flexibility of the bone; cracking of the bone; bones slipping out of position (particularly their ends); possible bruises near the location of the fracture; a tearing pain in the whole area of the fracture; insufficient function of the broken bone (e.g., instability of the adjacent joint).

When touched with some pressure the fracture is not always readily felt; the ever-present pain will get worse by touching and can lead to unconsciousness.

First action: cool the area of the broken bone with ethyl chloride, ice, water or moist dirt for at least 20 minutes. Avoid any further usage; send for a physician; put the broken bone on a level surface.

Entitled to help immediately: anybody.

Most qualified to give immediate help: first-aid personnel or physiotherapist, if present.

Immediate help: continue cold treatment; fix bone with the necessary materials (e.g., splint).

Most common mistakes in immediate help: heat treatment; attempts at motion; attempts to put bandages around injured area (danger of moving the ends of the broken bone) unless necessary to cover open wounds which occur at the same time.

Entitled to give further treatment: physician.

Most suitable place to provide further treatment: clinic specializing in orthopedic surgery.

Further treatment: according to recommendation of surgeon. The surgeon will normally x-ray the broken area and possibly operate to put the broken parts together. It will then be put in a cast or put out of use in a similar way. Physiotherapy will begin according to the speed of the healing process and the recommendation of the physician. The physiotherapy will be done according to kind and severity of the fracture and will consist of regenerating exercises, massages, and baths.

Further recommendations: check sites and implements for training and competition more thoroughly; in the case of *fatigue fractures:* train more on soft surfaces, wear shoes with more support; check diet to assure adequate intake of minerals (particularly calcium).

FROST BITE

Disturbances caused by exposing skin tissue too long to temperatures below freezing. The most common reasons for this disturbance are: too long an exposure; particularly of parts of the body which receive insufficient circulation (nose, chin, ears, fingers, toes) to sub-freezing temperatures; shoes and clothing which fit too tightly and got wet.

In the first stage all degrees of frost-bite look the same: white. The degree of frost-bite can often only be judged after two days. *1st degree:* white-colored skin followed by a reddening and swelling of the skin. *2nd degree:* dark red- or violet-colored skin, which feels numb and is blistered.

First action: swing around frost-bitten parts of the body to increase circulation by centrifugal force; keep the affected part of the body cool.

Entitled to help immediately: anybody.

Most qualified to give immediate help: anybody.

Immediate help: go to cool, dry room; get hot drinks; in the case of obvious 1st degree frost-bite: rub frost-bitten part with dry, rough sheets (e.g., towels) or walk bare-footed on rough carpet (for frost-bitten toes); keep constantly moving. In the case of 2nd degree burns: depending on the extent, send for physician.

Entitled to give further treatment: anybody.

Further treatment: try to warm up the frost-bitten part until the feeling comes back to the skin; this can be done most easily by taking a hot bath to warm the whole body. You should warm up so slowly, however, that the warming process is painless. In the case of 1st degree frost-bite use frost ointments.

In the case of 2nd degree frost-bite open up the blisters (blisters) and put dry sterile bandages on them; depending on their size you should see a physician before or after doing so.

Further recommendations: cover areas which are easily frost-bitten (e.g., ear muffs); use insolated clothing (particularly gloves and shoes); do not workout alone in severe cold—have have the exposed parts of the body regularly checked by a partner.

Frequent faults in treatment: faults in the immediate help; lack of medical check-up afterwards.

HEAT STROKE
Disturbance of the blood circulation due to insufficient heat release.

The most common reasons for this disturbance are: insufficient sweating in hot, humid weather; inability to sweat (e.g., low fluid level of the body); insufficient heat regulation as consequence of a general weakness of the body (e.g., infection, over-tiring, alcohol or nicotine excess).

The heat stroke is characterized by: its sudden occurrence, severe thirst, white or dark red color of the face, breathing difficulties, dry, covered tongue; hot skin, frequent collapse; the struck person loses balance, gives incoherent answers; possibility of cramps.

CAUTION: HEAT STROKE CAN BE LETHAL!

First action: go to cool, shady place immediately; put head on the same level as the body (possibly sideways—danger of vomiting).

Entitled to help immediately: anybody.

Most qualified to give immediate help: anybody

Immediate help: open clothing; rub temples, neck, and forehead with alcohol, eau de Cologne or other skin simulating substances to increase circulation of the head; cool compresses in the heart area; if necessary mouth-to-mouth breathing; send for physician.

51

Entitled to give further treatment: physician.

Further treatment: according to recommendations of physician.

Further recommendations: check salt intake and general physical condition; if athlete is over 40 have the degree of arthritis checked; check for hidden infections; when warming up in hot humid weather, take off sweat suit and wear sun hat; apply tanning lotion to head and neck against sun burn.

Frequent mistakes in treatment: covering body with material which does not let the heat of the body pass through; late treatment as the symptoms are not recognized as approaching heat stroke; keeping the head raised when lying down, or even the attempt to continue walking.

SUNSTROKE
Swelling of the brain by too much blood. The most common reasons for this disturbance are: too much sun on the unprotected head while not having enough activity at the same time. The indications are: dark red (blue) hot face; severe head ache; high pulse rate; sickness or even vomiting; dizziness; pressure on ears; unconsciousness.

First action: rest on cool, shady place with a raised position of the head.

Entitled to help immediately: anybody.

Most qualified to give immediate help: anybody.

Immediate help: open up tight fitting clothing; cool neck with ice, cold water or moist dirt; rubbing of the heart area; rest head and upper body in an elevated position; if necessary artificial (mouth-to-mouth) breathing; give some water (if unconscious, wait for this until consciousness returns); get transported to physician or hospital.

Frequent mistakes in the immediate help: head is not sufficiently raised (danger of suffocation when vomiting; danger of even more blood in the head); not staying with the affected person.

Entitled to give further treatment: physician.

Further treatment: according to recommendation of physician.

Further recommendations: cover head in time against sun even when running; aerobic training to increase capillarization and blood volume.

Frequent mistakes in treatment: late or insufficient care as the symptoms are not taken seriously enough.

STITCHES

Stitching, cramp-like pain over or under the lowest of the short ribs on the left or right or both sides. The most frequent reasons for this disturbance are: gas in the intestines, particularly in the upper left bend of the colon; cramps in the stomach muscles after running downhill or with a backward lean; spleen enlargement due to too much blood in it; stomach pain (lower edge) such as ingastritis or gastric ulcer; pain of the gall bladder, the liver or the bladder; cramps in the diaphragm or the stomach muscles; periostitis of the free ends of the 11th and 12th rib; cramps due to vegetative nerve disturbance; cold side wind; ulcers.

First action: continue workout or competition; try to relax painful area; inner relaxation by conscious deep breathing (change breath rhythm from the way you were breathing before); mechanical relaxation by strong, slow rubbing at the painful area; relax stomach muscles by leaning more forward; change rhythm and pace (sometimes running faster may help as much as running slower); if pain is unbearable stop workout; competition should not be ended unless pain makes it impossible.

Entitled to help immediately: anybody.

Most qualified to give immediate help: anybody.

Immediate help: rest in a quiet place, lying down sideways; cover with warm blanket; moist warm packing or hot water bottle on painful area; have some bisquits and camomile tea. If pain does not go away, go see physician at once; if stitches reappear at the very same spot frequently, see physician.

Frequent mistakes in the immediate help: taking circulation-stimulating substances (coffee, tea, nicotine, etc.); to see physician too late or not at all; eating something too heavy.

Entitled to give further treatment: physician.

Further treatment: according to recommendation of physician, who will normally run several checks to find or eliminate various possibilities for the stitch to reoccur.

Further recommendations: avoid fermented foods prior to workout, such as cabbage, legumes, sugar, fat or meat roasted in a lot of fat and food which is difficult to digest (such as hard boiled eggs, fruit with a hard skin); chew meals well; check everyday habits (you may need a lay-off to reduce general stress); check liquid input (you may need more to drink, but avoid alcohol and carbonated drinks); sleep more to relax; breathing exercises; avoid sports wear that fits too tight; in cold, windy weather protect the parts of the body which are exposed to the cold (e.g., newspaper under the running vest for road running competitions while facing the wind).

Frequent mistakes in treatment: superficial check-up; seeing physician too late.

INJURIES BY EVENT

(AND WHAT TO DO)

SPRINTS (100-200-400)

Traumatic problems

Pain in the back of the thigh

Reasons for pain: cramp; pull; beginning muscle rupture, muscle rupture.

Treatment: see under the above headings.

Hints for workouts: workouts do not need to be interrupted; there should be no sprinting, however, as long as the proper coordinated motion is hindered by the injury.

Compensatory workout: continue the normal weight training for sprinters for the upper body and arms but do not use injured muscles (e.g., benchpress, lifting while sitting, etc.).

Curing workouts: stimulate growth of injured muscle by isometric, slow isotonic or isokinetic resistance on machine or with partner. The following example has proven useful: while sitting on bench swing lower legs with weights attached. Lying on the stomach, lift lower legs against the isokinetic resistance of a partner into a vertical position.

Preventative workout: for exercises see curing workout; increase weight resistance; increase aerobic training for improved capillarization. Increase stretching exercises, e.g., reach for your toes while sitting and lean more and more forward.

Pain in the upper third of the front side of the thigh

Reasons for pain: muscle pull; beginning muscle rupture; muscle rupture.

Treatment: see under the above headings.

Hints for workouts: workouts do not need to be interrupted; there should be no sprinting, however, as long as the properly coordinated motion is hindered by the injury.

Compensatory workout: continue the normal weight training for sprinters for the upper body and arms, but do not use the injured muscles (e.g., benchpress, lifting while sitting).

Curing workouts: the following examples have proven useful: while sitting in the ground lift the straight legs slightly for up to 20 seconds, but avoid pain; sit-ups with slightly bent legs; sit-ups with weights behind the head; squats with increasing weight (on weight machine if available); make sure that the knees are straight on the squats and do not move sideways.

Preventative workouts: for exercises see curing workout; increase weight resistance; increase aerobic training for improved capillarization; stretching exercises, e.g., swing freely-extended leg from the hip while lying on a table; lie on stomach, reach for your ankles, and pull, causing a rocking motion; jump from a step (of increasing height) to the ground and directly up in the air for altitude or distance.

Technique-Related problems

Shin splints

Reasons for the pain: inflammation of the tendons and ligaments on the shin muscles and the periosteum of the shin.

Treatment: see under Inflammations, and especially periostitis.

Hints for workouts: workouts do not need to be interrupted but the running should be done on grass or any other soft and bouncing surface.

Supportive measures: fix the ankle joint at 90° angle by using inelastic tape for any workout involving running. Avoid carrying heavy weight in everyday life; no weight training which puts excessive weight on the legs.

Compensatory workouts: lie on your back and do bicycling in the air for up to 5 minutes (increase speed).

Curing workouts: continue compensative workouts and supportive measures.

Preventative workouts: wear properly designed shoes in everyday life and sport, with enough elasticity of the sole, soft upper leather and temperature insulation. Stretching exercises for the shin muscles, e.g., circles with your feet, squats with the heels on the ground; while sitting lift up and stretch out legs without touching ground with feet.

Pain in the bend of the knee

Reasons for the pain: inflamed bursae, tendons, tendon ends, and/or the back edges of the knee joint.

Treatment: see Inflammations, and especially of the bursa.

Hints for workouts: workouts do not need to be interrupted, but the running should be done on grass or any other soft and bouncing surface.

Supporting measures: avoid long fixations of the knee joint in the same position (e.g., long distance driving).

Compensatory workouts: lie on the ground and do bicycling in the air and shake legs repeatedly (up to 20 minutes).

Curing workouts: continue compensatory workouts; add aerobic running/jogging on soft ground.

Preventative workouts: for exercises, See Compensatory workouts; warm up very carefully before each workout; include stretching exercises for the back and the backs of both legs; loosen up arms and shoulder muscles one after the other and together with leg shaking.

Pain in the groin

Reasons for the pain: irritation or pull of the groin ligaments or the ligaments around the pelvis and adductor muscles.

Treatment: because of the closeness to the organs, the pain cannot be treated like a normal ligament pull as the ice treatment will lead to an inflammation of the bladder. Put on inelastic tape and an alcohol compress against the painful region. When chronic see Periostitis.

Hints for workouts: workouts do not need to be interrupted, but care should be taken not to do any long striding, side-stepping or bend running, since that will hurt. If pain is severe, nothing but weight training in a sitting or lying position can be done.

Pain in the shoulder-blade region

Reasons for the pain: mycosis, mycositis of the static shoulder muscles.

Treatment: see particularly under Inflammation of muscles.

Hints for workouts: workouts do not need to be interrupted, but weight training for the arms should be eliminated for a while.

Supportive measures: in everyday situations avoid typewriting, long driving (especially tight grip on the steering wheel); stressful situations; protect eyes against strong light; do not carry weights (e.g., a heavy bag).

Compensatory workouts: continue the normal sprint training but avoid the weight training for the arms.

Curing workouts: continue supportive measures and compensatory workouts.

Preventative workouts: hang by the hands on a ladder, lifting up the knees to the head while relaxing the back muscles; hang from head-high rings and swing the legs in a circular motion; turn the head in a full circular motion; turn the arms in a full circular motion; cross arms in front of your chest, putting hands on the opposite shoulders, then turn your head in a circular motion, nod, and pull shoulders down sideways.

MIDDLE DISTANCES (800-3000m)

Traumatic problems

Pain in the calves

Reasons for the pain: mycosis or inflammation of the static (holding) muscles; cramp or pull in the calf.

Treatment: see Inflammation of muscles, cramps, or muscle pull, respectively.

Hints for workouts: workouts do not need to be interrupted, but care should be taken to run at first only aerobically on soft surface (grass, with thick-soled shoes, etc.) in perfect coordination, to avoid compensatory pains (e.g., pains in the opposite knee because too much weight had been placed on it). In the case of a cramp or pull see measures under Muscle cramps or Muscle pull.

Supportive measures: active motion bath, e.g., hold tightly with both hands to the rim of a swimming pool and do an extensive crawl leg kick; when working out have inelastic tape around the ankle to relieve pain in the calf; increase salt, calcium and phosphorus intake.

Compensatory workouts: until pain is gone, you should have only aerobic workouts; in addition bicycle riding is possible.

Curing workouts: continue supportive measures and compensatory workouts.

Preventative workouts: when changing from road running to the track, from running flats to spikes, or in any other change of training sites and forms you should not change over abruptly but gently (first time you wear spikes after a long break, it should not be for more than 5 minutes). The adaptation to any new situation in the workouts should be done gently. Increase maximal weight on your shoulders—also on weight machine). Improve flexibility of your calf muscles (e.g., by leaning forward with straight body and heels on the ground against a wall 3 to 4 feet away); increase flexibility by exercising the ankles.

Technique-Related problems

Pains in the knees

Reasons for the pain: irritation of tendons, ligaments and/or periosta.

Treatment: see Inflammation of tendons and particularly Periostitis.

Hints for workouts: workouts do not need to be interrupted but care should be taken that workouts are done on soft, level ground (grass, soft soles of shoes); avoid monotonous pace (change pace).

Supportive measures: keep knee warm during the workout

by using sweat pants, knee warmers (mohair), analgesic balm (do not use heat ointment that only brings heat to the surface).

Compensatory workouts: if pains are so severe that running is not possible, go on a long, hard bicycle ride, at least as long as the workout would have taken.

Curing workouts: continue supportive measures and compensatory workouts.

Preventative workouts: when changing from road running onto the track, from running flats to spikes, or in any other case of change of training site or form you should not change over abruptly but gently (the first time you wear spikes again do not do so for more than 5 minutes). The adaptation to the new circumstances has to be slow and gentle. The flexibility of the calves, the thighs, the buttocks and back muscles has to be improved. This can be done by doing exercises, e.g., stand 3 to 4 feet away from wall, keep heels to the ground and lean gently forward against the wall; stand with straight legs and reach for your feet; lie on your back, stretch arms out sideways, and reach with a straight leg to the opposite hand; sit on ground with split legs and reach with your head to your knees and the floor between your legs; warm up more thoroughly before each workout, including more stretching.

Have an orthopedic check-up to see whether you have any congenital abnormalities (e.g., uneven leg length).

Work on full coordination to avoid any compensatory pain in the other leg while you still have the pain in the knee of the first one.

Open cuts from being spiked or falling down

Reasons for the pain: skin abrasions; open wounds; bruises; contusions; sprains.

Treatment: see under Abrasions, open wounds and Bruises and Contusions.

Hints for workouts: workouts do not need to be interrupted, but care should be taken that wound does not get freshly infected (apply bandages which do not hinder the functional motion) or re-open when moving and blood pressure is rising).

Supportive measures: bandages are to be fixed in such a way as to cover the wounds without hindering the functional motion.

Compensatory workouts: if the wound area is hindering the normal workout, one should do other circulation-intensive training, such as bicycle riding or weight training.

Curing workouts: continue supportive measures and compensatory workout.

Preventative workouts: train for dangerous situations such as running with other runners in a bunched group and deliberately change running rhythm; improve flexibility and reaction by team sports (such as basketball) or judo early in the season or off-season; work on tactics in your race preparation, including film material.

Unopened injuries from kicks, blows and bumps

Reasons for the pain: bruises or contusions.

Treatment: see *Bruises and Contusions.*

Hints for workouts: workouts do not need to be interrupted, but care should be taken, that the hurting muscles are not used for speed training (e.g., no sprint training if the legs are bruised).

Supportive measures: moist pressure-applying compress which does not hinder the workout.

Compensatory training: if the painful area hinders the functional motion of running, change to other exercises which are intensive on the circulatory system, such as bicycle riding, but which do not use the bruised muscles.

Curing workout: continue supportive measures and compensatory workouts.

Preventative workouts: train for dangerous situations such as group running with changing running rhythm; train flexibility and reaction by team sports (such as basketball) or judo in the early season or off-season; work on tactics in your race preparation including film material.

LONG DISTANCES (INCLUDING ROAD AND CROSS COUNTRY RUNNING)

Traumatic problems

Ankle pain

Reasons for the pain: inflammation of the joint.

Treatment: see *Inflammation of the Joint.*

Hints for workouts: workouts do not need to be interrupted, but on the first indications of pain, potential causes should be carefully investigated, such as: surface conditions (e.g., arched road, running on sloping beach with one foot always higher than the other); the shoes (pressure spots, uneven or worn down heels, etc.); orthopedic deformations (e.g., in the arch of the foot); or the way the foot is touching the ground when running.

Supportive measures: in case of *improper usage* of ankle, tape ankle in such a way that the functional, proper usage path of the ankle joint is still open, but no side motions are possible; continue workouts on perfectly level surface.

In the case of *over-training,* run on soft ground (preferably grass) and wear shoes with a thick, soft sole. If pains are very severe, do not run but do intensive bicycle riding instead.

Compensatory training: if the painful area is hindering the proper motion considerably, you should create a different workout which works as much on your circulatory system, but puts less weight on the ankles, e.g., bicycle riding, rowing, weightlifting (light weights, high repetitions).

Curing workout: continue supportive measures and compensatory workouts; include crawl swimming and walking in warm (preferably salt) water.

Preventative workouts: in case of improper usage strengthen foot and calf muscles, e.g., by grip exercises (lift towel or pieces of paper with your toes); do toe raises with weight on your back. In case of over-usage check training content and site; avoid workout and training site monotony.

Pain in the Achilles tendon

   Reasons for the pain: inflammation of the tendon.

   Treatment: see under *Inflammation of the Tendon.*

   Hints for workouts: see *Ankle Pain.*

   Supportive measures: see *Ankle Pain.*

   Compensatory workouts: see *Ankle Pain.*

   Curing workout: see *Ankle Pain.*

   Preventative workouts: see *Ankle Pain.* In the case of improper usage, make sure that you do not wear running shoes with heels that are too high or too narrow (danger of twisting the ankle); while sitting stretch out legs and arms at the same time, straight and parallel.

Technique-Related Problems

Pains in the arch of the foot

   Reasons for the pain: flat, splayfoot with falling or raising arches; periostitis; inflammation of the connective tissue; fatigue fracture.

Treatment: when the pain occurs and lasts for more than two workouts, see experienced orthopedist, who will x-ray the foot (possibility of fracture) or advise on arch support or other shoe inserts. To reduce pain see Inflammation of the joint.

Hints for workouts: workouts do not need to be interrupted, but carefully follow the advice of the orthopedist concerning the footwear and the shoe inserts.

Supportive measures: tight inelastic tape (about 1 inch wide) around the middle of the foot.

Compensatory workout: if the pain is so strong that proper running is impossible, change over to other training that is intensive on the circulary system (e.g., bicycle riding).

Curing workouts: strengthen foot muscles, e.g.: do grip exercises with the toes (lift towels); while standing on even surface pull towel (with a weight on the other end of it) with your toes underneath your feet; practice various toe positions as isometric exercises.

Preventative workouts: exercises as under curing workouts; jog occasionally bare-footed, at first for 15 minutes, then more.

Pain on top of the middle of the foot

Reasons for the pain: periostitis; inflammation of the tendons; fatigue fracture.

Treatment: when pains appear see experienced orthopedist, who might x-ray the foot for possible fracture. To reduce pain, see under Periostitis.

Hints for workouts: workouts do not need to be interrupted, but care should be taken that the training takes place on soft level ground, preferably on grass; have soft soles of running shoes, soft upper leather and protection against rubbing of the shoe laces. Avoid jumping exercises.

65

Supportive measures: support foot with unelastic tape to avoid painful movements.

Compensatory workouts: see *Ankle Pain.*

Curing workouts: continuation of compensatory workouts and supportive measures.

Preventative workouts: see *Pains in the Arch of the Foot.*

Pains in the hip

Reasons for the pain: inflammation of the joint; periostitis; irritation and/or inflammation of muscles.

Treatment: x-ray control by experienced orthopedist, to check for in-born abnormalities of the hip and pelvis region, which will cause pain with increased workout load. If this is not the case, see Periostitis.

Inflammation of the joint and Inflammation of muscles

Hints for workouts: the workouts do not need to be interrupted, but the orthopedic control is absolutely necessary (possible difficulties later on if neglected). Avoid jumping and similar bouncing exercises. Work on good coordination, as pain may be the compensatory result of some other ailment.

Supportive measures: wear elastic tight-fitting pressure bandages around hip (rubber pants) and abdomen.

Compensatory workout: if the painful area is hindering the proper running motion considerably, do a different workout which is active on the circulatory system (e.g., bicycle riding with little resistance but high speed; swimming).

Curing workout: if not recommended differently by orthopedist, continue supportive measures and compensatory workouts.

Preventative workouts: strengthening of hip and thigh

muscles by exercises such as the following: (1) while standing put a book between your knees and press it isometrically as hard as you can for 10 seconds (repeat); sitting upright, knees together, cross arms and push your knees apart with your hands against maximal resistance of your adductor muscles; then close the knees against the resistance of your hands (isokinetic strength training for your adductor muscles); (2) while sitting in a hurdling position with your right foot out in front change to your left foot in front without the help of your arms or hands; duck walk with bended knees (possibly with weight on your shoulders).

Back Pain

Reasons for the pain: sciatic inflammation; damaged disc; inflammation of the muscles; inflammation of the joints.

Treatment: x-ray control by an experienced orthopedist; if no abnormalities of the spine are to be found see Inflammation of sciatic nerve.

Hints for workouts: the workouts do not need to be interrupted, but the orthopedic control is absolutely necessary (possible difficulties later on if neglected); avoid jumping and similar bouncing exercises; avoid leaning forward or backward. Do not carry weights or even heavy bags in everyday life and do not sit in a bent position for any length of time.

Supportive measures: in everyday situation and workouts wear mohair underwear which covers the painful area; wear woolen knee and foot covers, to make sure that from there no cold can be passed on to the groin; it may be necessary to protect the groin by a heavy leather weight lifter belt.

Compensatory workouts: do your running on soft ground, grass, wood paths, etc., and wear shoes with soft sole.

Curing workouts: if not advised otherwise by orthopedist, continue supportive measures and compensatory workouts.

Preventative workouts: strengthening of the long and short neck and back muscles; e.g., standing with your feet one ft. away from a wall, press with your whole back isometrically against it with a straight back; lie face down on a bench so that your upper body extends past the bench, have the feet held by someone, and place weight on your neck; raise the upper body, remain free in the air for 10 seconds, then move slowly down; same position, but have arms extended with weights or heavy ball in your hands and do circles with your upper body; lie on the ground with closed legs, arms on your stomach, lift and hold your hip as high in the air as possible for 10 seconds.

HURDLES AND STEEPLECHASE

Traumatic problems

Pains in the Ankle

Reasons for the pain: inflammation of the joint; rupture of synovial joint; periostitis; pulled tendons; inflammation of tendons.

Treatment: inflammation of the joint; periostitis; pulled tendons, inflammation of tendons.

Hints for workouts: the workouts do not need to be interrupted, but you should not hurdle for some time; avoid jumping exercises.

Supportive measures: secure the foot in a right-angle position by taping up to the shin.

Compensatory workouts: include extended exercises on one hurdle to compensate for the lay-off. Do sprints without hurdles (or steeplechasing at race pace without hurdles), if this can be done painlessly.

Curing workouts: continue compensatory workouts and supportive measures.

Preventative workouts: improve hurdling technique; improve strength of the lower part of the leg: e.g., jumps from an elevated position to the ground then up again as far or as high as possible (possibly with weights on the neck); jumping over hurdles or on staircase; do toe raises while standing with a heavy weight on shoulders.

Pains in the Bend of the Knee

Reasons for the pain: inflammation of the bursa, the tendons or ends of tendons; pull of ligaments.

Treatment: see *inflammation of bursa, inflammation of tendons, pull of ligaments.*

Hints for workouts: the workouts do not need to be interrupted, but you should avoid running over hurdles if the pain hinders well coordinated, proper motion.

Supportive measures: keep knee joint warm on all sides with a mohair cover.

Compensatory workouts: take hurdles or steeples only if this can be done painlessly. Continue with the running workouts, but look for soft ground (grass) and wear shoes with soft soles.

Curing workouts: continue compensatory workouts and supportive measures.

Preventative workouts: to strengthen muscles of the knee area, e.g., hang by the hands on an exercise ladder, face the ladder, and with weights attached, raise and lower the legs (from the knee down), and then let them hang freely; lie on stomach, raise the lower legs against the isokinetic resistance of a partner, then bring them down against the same isokinetic resistance; workout isotonically on weight machine for the lower legs, and isometrically at all possible angles of the knee joint.

Pains in the Groin

Reasons for the pain: irritation or pull of the ligaments in the groin, the ends of tendons at the hip or the beginning of the adductor muscles.

Treatment: because of the proximity of the organs the pain cannot be treated like a pull (danger of inflamed bladder from cold treatment); wrap with a layer of inelastic tape, which presses an alcohol compress against the painful area. If the pain is chronic treat like periostitis.

Hints for the workouts: the workouts do not need to be interrupted, but you should avoid running over hurdles, if this cannot be done without pain and with good coordination (danger of compensatory injury).

Supportive measures: have elastic pressure bandages (e.g., rubber pants) around hip including the upper part of the thighs.

Compensatory workouts: take hurdles only if this can be done painlessly. Continue with the running workouts, but on soft ground (grass) and with shoes with soft soles.

Curing workouts: continue compensatory workouts and supportive measures; in addition you should go to a swimming pool and do breaststroke swimming or hold on to the edge of the pool and do the breaststroke kick in the water.

Preventative workouts: increased flexibility workouts for the hip area, which should not be left out in any warm-up program and should slowly be increased. Examples: stand upright, lift one leg, hold knee and make circular motions with the knee; stand upright, raise one leg to an elevated support (e.g., hurdle) reach to the ground with hands, then bend slowly backward with the opposite foot flat on the floor, make circular motions with the whole upper body. Lie on the ground, bring knee of one leg to chin, hold it with the arms, and move the leg slowly isokinetically sideways against the resistance of your arm; sit on floor with crossed legs, hold knees with the opposite hands, close knees against isokinetic resistance of the hands, then open knees against isokinetic resistance of hands to work on the adductors.

Pains in the Buttock Muscles

Reasons for the pain: irritation, pull or inflammation of the tendons at the end of the biceps femoris near the caput longum of the tuber ischiadicum *(see illustration)*

Treatment: see *Pulled Tendons.*

Hints for workouts: the workouts do not need to be interrupted, but you should not run over hurdles as long as the well coordinated motion is hindered by pain.

Supportive measures: elastic rubber bandage around thigh which should reach far enough that it relieves some of the pressure from the tendon and holds the painful area together.

Compensatory workouts: run over hurdles only when pain free to avoid compensatory injuries elsewhere. For your customary running workouts use soft level ground (grass) and soft-soled shoes.

Curing workouts: continue compensatory measures and supportive workouts; in addition, swim or at least do the crawl motion with your legs at the edge of the pool.

Preventative workouts: increased exercises to stretch and strengthen thigh and hip muscles. Examples: while sitting in the hurdling position with left leg forward, change to the right leg forward without the help of your hands; sit on the floor with your legs spread as far as you can, move your upper body down to one knee, then to the other, then to the floor; lie on your back, lift your legs straight, bring them down slowly isometrically and isokinetically against the resistance of a partner or isotonically against the resistance of a weight machine; lie on your back, lift legs and neck, and do a rocking motion on your back.

Technique-related problems

Bruised Heel

Reasons for the pain: bruises of the calcaneus, periostitis of the heel.

Treatment: in acute cases see *Bruises and Contusions;* in chronic condition see *Periostitis.*

Hints for workouts: the workouts do not need to be interrupted but you should not run over hurdles if the pain hinders the well-coordinated motion.

Supportive measures: the heel should be protected with either foam rubber underneath or a nylon cup.

Compensatory workouts: run over hurdles only when painfree. Avoid any exercises in which you land on the heel (e.g., jumping). Continue running workouts on soft surface (grass) and with soft-soled shoes.

Curing workouts: continue supportive measures and compensatory workouts, go to swimming pool (or preferably the ocean) and do crawl kick in the (salt) water.

Preventative workouts: improvement of the hurdling technique and the basic speed; strengthening of the adductor muscles, particularly of the trail leg; improvement of the flexibility of the hip and buttock muscles: e.g., sit in hurdling position and move—without the help of your hands—to the opposite leg extended; in standing position, circle knee with and without resistance of your arm; sit with crossed pulled-up legs, open and close knees against the resistance of the opposite arms (crossed arm position), both isokinetically and isometrically; while standing, put trailing leg on box or hurdle, pull in trailing position against resistance of rubber band or partner.

Back Pain

Reasons for the pain: irritation or pull of the back muscles or of the ligaments of the spine.

Treatment: because of the proximity of the organs the injury cannot be treated like a pull; wear inelastic taping (apply in exhaled position) around the respective part of the body under which alcohol compresses can be attached; fango packings; hot salt bandages and salt compresses; when pain is no longer acute, massage.

Hints for workouts: workouts do not need to be interrupted but care should be taken not to run over hurdles while the pain hinders the properly coordinated motion.

Supportive measures: even when taking up hurdling again the taping should be kept on for some time.

Compensatory workouts: run over hurdles only if this motion can be done without pain to avoid compensatory pain elsewhere. The amount of running depends on how much can be handled without an increase in pain.

Curing workouts: continue supportive measures and compensatory workouts and include stretching and bending of the body, such as: lie on your back on the ground, lift your knees to the chin, and do rocking motion.

Preventative workouts: improvement of the flexibility of all the back muscles by exercises such as: sitting on the ground with crossed legs, move with your body forward between the legs and over each leg; lie on the ground, stretching arms out shoulder high, swing the extended legs from one hand to the other, without touching them; circling with your hips.

SHOT PUT AND DISCUS

Traumatic problems

Pain in the Metacarpophalangea Joint (between palm and fingers)

Reasons for the pain: pull of tendons, ligaments and joint.

Treatment: see particularly *Pulls of Ligaments.*

Hints for workouts: the workouts need not be interrupted but you should avoid throwing or weight exercises in which your fingers hold with a tight grip or are extended fully.

Supportive measures: attach fingers to palm in the least painful position with a tight fitting adhesive tape.

Compensatory workouts: particularly weight training on weight machines where the weight can rest on the palms and need not be held by the fingers.

Curing workouts: continue supportive measures and compensatory workouts; include isometric and isokinetic exercises for the improvement of strength and circulation of the palm and finger muscles; e.g., hold a tennis ball and press it together with the tips of the fingers; put the palms and finger tips of the hands together and press them isometrically and isokinetically, moving one against the other with all your strength; rapid opening and closing of your hands and spreading of your fingers.

Prophylactic workouts: strengthen your hands and fingers with exercises from the curing workouts; further examples are: push-ups on your finger tips; adding hand-claps in mid-air; pull ups on your front finger joints.

Technique-related problems

Ankle Pains

Reasons for the pains: pulls of tendons, ligaments, or joint; periostitis.

Treatment: in acute cases see particularly *Pulls of Ligaments.* In chronic condition particularly *Periostitis.*

Hints for workouts: the workouts do not need to be

74

interrupted, but you should not throw (danger of faulty technique caused by avoiding painful positions) or weight lift with pressure on your ankles (no squats).

Supportive measures: in all weight and throwing workouts you should have your ankle taped in the least painful position.

Compensatory workouts: weight exercises on machine where ankles are not burdened (e.g., bench press).

Curing workouts: continue supportive measures and compensatory workouts but include in addition exercises for more strength and circulation of the ankle joint area, e.g., toe gripping exercises (lift pieces of paper or towels, etc., with your toes); circle your feet against the resistance of your hands; do the crawl kick in the swimming pool while holding on to the edge of the pool.

Preventative workouts: strengthen the ankle with intensified exercises of the curing workouts. Further exercises: toe lifts; raise and stand on the inner or outer rim of your feet with or without weights (can also be done on weight machine); jump from platform or box and up again as high (or as far) as you can.

Pains in the Groin

Reasons for the pains: irritation or pull of tendons or muscles in the adductor region; irritation or inflammation of periosteum; hernia (rupture in the groin).

Treatment: see experienced surgeon who will examine for hernia. Because of the proximity of the organs the pains can not be treated like a pull, as the cold treatment will result in an inflammation of the bladder. Put on inelastic tape which presses an alcohol compress against the painful region. Sit in clay, salt, or ichthyol bath.

Hints for workouts: the workouts do not need to be interrupted but you should avoid throwing and weight training which causes the groin to hurt.

Supportive measures: in workouts and everyday situations wear elastic tight-fitting taping or rubber pants which press together the whole abdominal area, including the thighs.

Compensatory workouts: weight training in which the painful area is not used.

Curing workouts: continue supportive measures and compensatory workouts and include isometric and isokinetic exercises to strengthen and improve circulation in the whole adductor area; sit with crossed legs, open and close legs isokinetically against the resistance of the crossed arms; stand, put tennis ball between your knees, press it tightly together.

Preventative workouts: improvement of strength and flexibility in the adductor region by exercises of the curing workouts; further examples: sit in hurdling position, change from one forward leg to the other without the assistance of your hands; general hurdling exercises.

Pains in the Chest Muscles

Reasons for the pains: irritation or pull of the chest muscles (pectoralis major, pectoralis minor).

Treatment: see particularly *Muscle Pull.*

Hints for workouts: the workouts do not need to be interrupted but you should avoid exercises such as discus throwing by which the pectoralis muscles are stretched.

Supportive measures: elastic bandages over the whole chest.

Compensatory workouts: primarily weight training by which the painful muscles are not used.

Curing workouts: isometric and isokinetic exercises to strengthen the chest muscles. Example: put palms together in front of your chest and press isometrically in various positions (10 seconds in each).

Preventative workouts: improvement of strength and flexibility by increased exercises of the curing workouts. Further examples: push ups with hand clapping in mid-air; handstand at wall with various arm widths, push-ups; discus throwing with women's shot; putting with over-weight shot.

JAVELIN

Traumatic problems

Pains in the Knee Joint

Reasons for the pains: irritation, pull or inflammation of the tendons, ligaments or periosteum in the knee area.

Treatment: an experienced orthopedist should check for miniscus injuries. In chronic condition see *Periostitis;* in acute cases *Ligament Pulls.*

Hints for workouts: workouts do not need to be interrupted but you should avoid throwing with full run-up where the knee is burdened again.

Supportive measures: keep painful area warm at all times with mohair knee bandages.

Compensatory workouts: primarily weight training, without using the painful area.

Curing workouts: continue supportive measures and compensatory workouts; include crawl kick in (salt water) pool.

Preventative workouts: improvement of the strength of the whole legs to increase stability at the knee joint; improvement of coordination of the whole leg by: aerobic jogging; jumping up and down from knee-high platform with sand bag or weights on the shoulders; lying on stomach, raising and lowering of the lower legs against the isokinetic resistance of a partner; toe raises, without and then with weights (also possible on weight machine).

Back Pain

Reasons for the pains: irritation or pull of the muscle, tendons, ligaments in the back or of the discs of the spine.

Treatment: an experienced orthopedist should check whether the discs are injured. Because of the closeness of the organs the injury cannot be treated like a pull, as the cold treatment would create an inflammation. Put on corset or inelastic taping (applied in an exhaled position) under which you should apply alcohol compresses; fango packings; hot salt packings or hot salt water baths; when pain has decreased, massages; inflammation reduction by ABC-plaster or ichthyol ointment.

Hints for workouts: the workouts do not need to be interrupted but you should be careful not to throw as long as the pain is hindering well-coordinated motion.

Supportive measures: after having started throwing again the corset or chest taping should be continued for some time.

Compensatory workouts: aerobic jogging; weight training by which the painful area is not included.

Curing workouts: continue supportive measures and compensatory workouts including exercises to strengthen the whole upper body, such as: sitting on floor, slow sit-ups at first isometrically holding at various positions, then isokinetically pressing against the resistance of a partner on the way up and down.

Preventative workouts: improvement of flexibility and strength of the whole back area by exercises such as: lie on stomach, hold arms out with medicine ball or light shot, then raise upper body and throw forward; lie on back, raise your body to high arch on hands and feet, then lift yourself up from arched position to standing on feet or hands; hang from horizontal bar, over head-height, place heavy ball 3 feet behind you, swing backward and then on the way forward, kick it—with both feet swinging—as far forward as you can.

Pains in the Elbow

Reasons for the pains: inflammation of the tendons, joints, ligaments, periostea, bursae or motor nerves; pull of the tendons or ligaments; comminuted fracture; rupture of cartilage.

Treatment: an experienced orthopedist or surgeon should check whether bone or cartilage is injured. In other acute cases see particularly *Pull of Ligaments;* in chronic conditions see *Periostitis.*

Hints for workouts: workouts do not need to be interrupted, but you should avoid throwing while the pain is hindering the proper well-coordinated motion.

Supportive measures: keep the painful area warm by mohair elbow cap.

Compensatory workouts: aerobic running; weight training by which the elbow is not burdened.

Curing workouts: continue supportive measures and compensatory workouts, include coordination exercises, stretching and strengthening of the arm and shoulder region by exercises such as: attach legs on rim of (salt water) swimming pool, do the crawl arm motion; isometric and isokinetic arm exercises against own body or partner, such as pushing hands together in various positions in front of the chest and shift positions of maximal pressure on both hands against each other.

Preventative workouts: exercises as in curing workouts; in addition, isotonic exercises such as push-ups with inward-pointing fingers; walk on your hands (pointed inward), with partner supporting your feet; hand stand against wall (inward-pointing fingers); push-ups.

Technique-related problems

Pains in the Shoulder Area

Reasons for the pains: irritation or pull of tendons, ligaments or cartilages; rupture of cartilage or bone; periostitis.

Treatment: an experienced orthopedist or surgeon should check whether bone or cartilage is injured. In other acute cases see particularly Pull of ligaments. In chronic condition see Periostitis.

Hints for workouts: the workouts do not need to be interrupted, but you should avoid throwing as long as the pain is hindering the proper and well-coordinated motion.

Supportive measures: have inelastic tape put on which allows for functionally proper javelin-throwing, but which stops side motions.

Compensatory workouts: bicycle riding; weight training by which the painful area is not being used.

Curing workouts: continue supportive measures and compensatory workouts but include exercises for the improved coordination, flexibility and strengthening of the shoulder area, such as: put feet on rim of swimming pool and do the arm motion of all swimming strokes in the water; arm circles, isokinetically against the resistance of a partner.

Preventative workout: exercises as in the curing workouts and in addition isotonic exercises for the shoulders, such as: pull-ups; swinging and circling on horizontal bar; push-ups off the ground (when coming down you should move your hands from an inward position to one more and more outward and back); push-ups, leaving the ground and landing each time with the hands further apart.

Pains in the Neck Area

Reasons for the pains: irritation or pull of the neck

muscles, injured discs; periostitis.

Treatment: an experienced orthopedist or surgeon should check whether a bone or disc is injured. In other acute cases see particularly *Muscle Pulls;* in chronic condition particularly *Periostitis.*

Hints for workouts: workouts do not need to be interrupted; extreme care in throwing since the pain may hinder the proper motion.

Supportive measures: inelastic tape pressing felt or alcohol compress against the painful area.

Compensatory workouts: bicycle riding; exercises where the pain does not appear (e.g., bench pressing).

Curing workouts: continue compensatory workouts and supportive measures and include increased coordination, flexibility and strength training for the neck area, such as: circle your head; drop your head forward, backward, and sideward and let it swing freely; place head in various positions and isometrically contract neck muscles; circling your head isokinetically against the resistance of your hands (press your head backward, in particular).

Preventative workouts: exercises as in curing workouts but include now isotonic exercises for the neck, such as hammer throwing (with well stretched arms); bowling.

HAMMER

Traumatic problems

Pains in the Knees

Reasons for the pains: irritation or pull of the tendons or ligaments in the knee area; meniscus problems.

Treatment: an experienced orthopedist should check whether the meniscus is injured. In other acute cases see particularly *Ligament Pulls* and in chronic condition particularly *Periostitis.*

Hints for the workouts: workouts do not need to be interrupted, but you should not circle with the hammer, throw after turning, nor do any other exercises which burden the knee.

Supportive measures: inelastic tape (possibly you should put a felt or an alcohol compress underneath).

Compensatory workouts: particularly weight training which does not burden the knees.

Curing workouts: continue compensatory workouts and supportive measures; in addition do strengthening exercises such as: holding on to rim of a pool, do the crawl kick in the water.

Preventative workouts: increase the strength of the whole leg to minimize the twisting burden on the knee with exercises such as: aerobic jogging; jump up to and down from a knee-high platform with weights on your shoulders; bicycle riding (uphill) against severe resistance; stand with weights on the neck and do toe raises on inner and outer rims of feet.

Pains in Groin

Reasons for the pains: irritation or pull of the muscles or tendons in the adductor region; periostitis; hernia (rupture of the groin).

Treatment: see an experienced surgeon who will examine for hernia. Because of the proximity of the organs the pains cannot be treated like a pull, as the cold treatment will result in an inflammation of the bladder or other organs. Apply alcohol compress which is held tightly against the painful region with unelastic tape. In chronic condition see *Periostitis.*

Hints for workouts: the workouts do not need to be interrupted but you should not throw the hammer and should avoid leg positions in which the pain reoccurs (e.g., spreading and twisting of legs).

Supportive measures: in workouts and everyday life wear elastic taping or rubber pants over the whole painful area, including the thighs.

Compensatory workouts: bicycle riding; weight training in which the painful area is not being used.

Curing workouts: continue supportive measures and compensatory workouts; in addition include isometric and isokinetic exercises for the adductor region, such as: hold with hands on rim of pool and do the breast stroke kick in the water; sit with crossed legs, open and close knees isometrically and isokinetically against the resistance of the hands; press tennis ball between your knees together as hard as you can.

Preventative workouts: improvement of leg strength and flexibility particularly of the adductor muscles by exercises such as those under the curing workouts; other examples are: sit in hurdling position and change lead leg without the use of your hands; then carry weight on your shoulders while doing so; duck walk with and without weights on your shoulders; general hurdling exercises; sit with crossed legs, pressing with your one foot against the inside of the opposite leg, and move with isokinetic pressure through the full range of motion.

Technique-related problems

Pains in the Ankle

Reasons for the pains: pull of tendons, ligaments or joint; periostitis.

Treatment: in acute cases see particularly *Ligament Pull;* in chronic condition particularly *Periostitis.*

Hints for workouts: the workouts do not need to be

interrupted but you should not throw the hammer and should avoid weight training that puts pressure on either foot.

Supportive measures: in all workouts you should tape the ankle in the least painful position.

Compensatory workouts: particularly weight training and training on the weight machine, whereby the ankles are not burdened.

Curing workouts: continue supportive measures and compensatory workouts and include isometric and isokinetic exercises to strengthen the ankle joints and improve circulation in the whole area, e.g., toe gripping (lift pieces of paper, towels, etc.); circle, stretch and flex feet against the resistance of your hands; hold on to rim of swimming pool and do the crawl kick in the water.

Preventative workouts: strengthen the ankle area by intensifying the curing workouts and further exercises such as: standing with weights on your shoulders, raise to ball, heel, and both rims of your feet; stand with weights on your shoulders, knees slightly bent, and jump in semi-circles; maximal 10-yard sprints out of blocks.

LONG JUMP AND TRIPLE JUMP

Traumatic problems

Pains in the Knee Area

Reasons for the pains: irritation, pull or inflammation of tendons, bursae, ends of bones or periosta in the knee area.

Treatment: have experienced orthopedist check whether the meniscus is injured. In other acute cases see particularly *Ligament Pull,* and in chronic condition *Periostitis.*

Hints for workouts: do not interrupt the workouts but do not jump or do other exercises which burden the knee joint.

Supportive measures: attach 1 inch tape tightly around the lower edge of knee; keep painful area warm with mohair knee cap.

Compensatory workouts: particularly weight training by which the painful area is not used.

Curing workouts: continue supportive measures and compensatory workouts; in addition, do the crawl kick in a pool, holding with your hands to the rim.

Preventative workouts: increase the stability of your stand by coordination and strengthening exercises for the whole chain of muscles in the legs by exercises such as: aerobic jogging; lie on stomach, lift and straighten lower legs against the isokinetic resistance of a partner; jump from step down to the ground and immediately as high in the air again as possible; sit on the ground, stretch out legs, place weight or sand bag on your feet, raise and lower feet.

Pains on the Front Side of the Thighs

Reasons for the pains: irritation, pull or beginning rupture in the region of the quadriceps femoris.

Treatment: see *Muscle Pull and Muscle Rupture.*

Hints for workouts: workouts do not need to be interrupted but you should avoid long jumping and exercises in which the quadriceps femoris is particularly used.

Supportive measures: inelastic tape around the painful area.

Compensatory workouts: particularly weight training in which the painful area is not involved.

Curing workouts: continue supportive measures and

compensatory workouts and further exercises such as crawl kick in swimming pool; sitting on ground without hands on the floor, raise straight legs for 20 seconds; put light weight on feet and raise straight legs; lie on back, raise thighs against the isokinetic resistance of your hands on your knees.

Preventative workouts: continue exercises as under curing workouts; stretching exercises; exercises for the improvement of the capillarization such as aerobic running; swing a wide figure eight with one leg while standing on the other; sit-ups with weight behind the neck and bended knees; lying on stomach, raise and lower the lower legs against the isokinetic resistance of a partner; jump with both legs high in the air and kick your buttocks with your heels.

Technique-related problems

Bruised Heel

Reasons for the pains: bruises or inflammation (periostitis) of the heel.

Treatment: in acute cases see particularly *Bruises and Contusions;* in chronic condition see *Periostitis.*

Hints for workouts: workouts do not need to be interrupted but you should not jump while the pain is hindering the proper coordinated motion.

Supportive measures: the heel should be protected either with foam rubber or a nylon cup.

Compensatory workouts: running on soft ground; weight training which doesn't put weight on the heel.

Curing workouts: continue supportive measures and compensatory workouts and include exercises for the painful region for better circulation such as crawl kick in a pool.

Preventative workouts: improve your jumping technique.

Pains in the Ankles

86

Reasons for the pains: irritation, pull or inflammation of muscles, tendons, ligaments, periosta or the joint in the ankle.

Treatment: in acute cases see particularly *Pulled Ligaments;* in chronic condition *Periostitis.*

Hints for workouts: workouts do not need to be interrupted but you should not jump or do weight training which puts strain on your ankles.

Supportive measures: fix ankle with an inelastic taping in the position which is the least painful before any workout.

Compensatory workouts: particularly weight training by which the ankles are not burdened.

Curing workouts: continue supportive measures and compensatory workouts and include isometric and isokinetic exercises to strengthen the ankle region and foot muscles by lifting towels or pieces of paper with your bare toes; ankle circling, stretching and flexing against the isokinetic resistance of your hands; crawl kick in (salt water) pool.

Preventative workouts: improvement of the strength of the ankle joint by intensifying the exercises of the curing workouts and further examples such as to raise and lower yourself from flat feet to your toes; repeat on inner and the outer edges of your feet with a heavy weight on your shoulders (also on weight machine); aerobic running; while sitting, flex your feet against the isokinetic resistance of your hands.

Back Pain

Reasons for the pain: jolting or pull of the back muscles or discs.

Treatment: have an experienced orthopedist check whether the spine or discs are injured. Because of the closeness of the organs the injury cannot be treated like a pull, as the cold treatment will cause inflammation of kidneys, etc. Have inelastic taping or corset put on (in exhaled position) over alcohol compresses attached to the painful area; fango packings; hot salt water packings; when pain is no longer acute, local massage.

Hints for workouts: the workouts do not need to be interrupted but you should not jump or do stretching exercises for the back while the pain is hindering proper coordination.

Supportive measures: after the jumping in workouts has started again you should continue for some time to wear the corset or taping.

Compensatory workouts: jumping, running, exercising with reduced intensity for the back region.

Curing workouts: continue supportive measures and compensatory workouts. Include flexing and stretching upper body against resistance, e.g., lie on stomach, raise arms, raise upper body against the isokinetic resistance of a partner and isometrically hold at various angles for 10 seconds each; stand, lean forward, swing weights with your arms (start with 10 pounds and increase); lie on stomach, raise and lower legs and upper body.

Preventative workouts: strengthening of all back muscles by exercises such as: lying on stomach, hold medicine ball (or light shot) in both hands, raise upper body and extend arms and throw ball as far as you can; aerobic running; hang from high horizontal bar, reach for medicine ball two feet behind you with extended feet, hold ball between your feet, and swing forward in a kicking motion, to throw the ball as far forward as possible; lie on back, raise and lower your hips (with and without resistance of a partner) without the usage of your hands.

HIGH JUMP

Traumatic Problems

Pains in the Knee

Reasons for the pains: irritation, pull or rupture of tendons or ligaments; inflammation of bursae, ends of bone or periosta in the knee region.

Treatment: an experienced orthopedist should check whether the meniscus or knee-cap is injured. In acute cases see particularly *Ligament Pull* and *Inflammation of Bursa;* in chronic condition particularly *Periostitis.*

Hints for workouts: workouts do not need to be interrupted but you should not jump or do exercises whereby weight is put on the knee.

Supportive measures: put one-inch tape tightly around the lower edge of your knee; keep knee warm with a mohair cover.

Compensatory workouts: particularly weight training by which the painful area is not being used.

Curing workouts: continue supportive measures and compensatory workouts and include crawl kick in pool.

Preventative workouts: strengthening of the thigh muscles by exercises such as: sprinting; lying on stomach, raise legs to your back and then lower them diagonally against the isokinetic resistance of a partner; press isometrically backward against resistance of partner; sit-ups (with crossed legs) with and without weights behind your neck.

Technique-related problems

Pains in the Groin

Reasons for the pain: irritation or pull of groin ligaments,

ligaments of the pelvis or ligaments in the adductor region.

Treatment: because of the proximity of the organs the injury cannot be treated like a pull with cold treatment (risk of an inflamed bladder); put on inelastic taping which presses an alcohol compress against the painful region. In chronic condition see particularly *Periostitis.*

Hints for workouts: the workouts do not need to be interrupted, but you should avoid high jumping and exercises in which you spread your legs to such an extent that it will be painful for the involved area.

Supportive measures: put 1-inch tape around waist just above the upper end of the thighs.

Compensatory workouts: avoid jumping while it is painful as this may negatively influence your coordination; avoid other exercises which are painful for the region; aerobic running on soft ground; weight training which does not burden the groin.

Curing workouts: continue supportive measures and compensatory workouts; include the breast stroke kick in salt water or swimming pool.

Preventative workouts: improvement of flexibility and strengthening of the leg muscles by exercises such as: sitting in hurdle position, shift the other leg forward without using your hands; do the same while carrying weight in each hand; sit, cross your legs, open and close them against the isokinetic resistance of your arms; hang from chest-high horizontal bar in one knee bend, kick heavy ball forward with extended leg from a position two feet behind the body.

POLE VAULT

Traumatic problems

Reasons for the pains: irritation or pull of muscles, tendons or ligaments, possibly slipped disc.

Treatment: an experienced orthopedist should check for spine or disc trouble; because of the closeness of the organs it cannot be treated like a pull as the cold treatment will cause inflammation (e.g., of the kidneys); you should wear a corset or inelastic taping (fixed in exhaled position) with alcohol compresses underneath; fango packings; hot salt (water) packings; after the pain is no longer acute, massage; in chronic condition see Inflammation of the joints.

Hints for workouts: the workouts do not need to be interrupted but you should not jump while the pain is hindering the proper motion.

Supportive measures: after jumping has been resumed the corset should be worn for a few more weeks.

Compensatory workouts: aerobic running; weight training whereby the painful area is not being used.

Curing workouts: continue supportive measures and compensatory workouts and other exercises to strengthen the torso, such as: sit-ups against the isokinetic resistance of a partner; sit-ups isometrically held at various positions; lie on bench on your stomach, hold upper body extending over the edge of the bench, and medicine ball in extended arms.

Preventative workouts: improvement of run-up and jumping technique, strengthening of upper arm and back muscles by exercises such as: bench press; slow arm flexions against weight resistance; maximal resistance expander (metal springs with handle bars on each side) in front of body, right handed athlete pulls with the right hand and pushes with the left (left handed vice versa); flop jumping; while hanging from (reach high) horizontal bar, take heavy ball between your ankles and swing from a backward position to a forward position, releasing it with a strong kicking motion; increase weight of curing workouts.

Technique-related problems

Pains in the Lower Arm

Reasons for the pain: irritation, inflammation or pull of tendons, muscles, periosta or ligaments in the lower arm.

Treatment in acute cases see particularly *Muscle Pull;* in chronic condition see *Periostitis.*

Hints for workouts: the workouts do not need to be interrupted but you should not do any vaulting while the pain is hindering the well-coordinated motion.

Supportive measures: put un elastic tape around the whole lower arm with alcohol compress directly on the painful area.

Compensatory workouts: sprint training; aerobic running.

Curing workouts: continue supportive measures and compensatory workouts and include exercises to loosen up and strengthen the arm muscles, such as: fix feet at the rim of a swimming pool and practice arm actions of all swim strokes; put hands together and press isokinetically at all possible angles and heights; hold weights in each hand and swing in all directions.

Preventative workouts: intensify curing workouts; include exercises at the horizontal bar (pull ups, turns, etc.); boxing with sand bag or punching bag; handstand push-ups against wall or with partner; hammer throwing.

REFERENCES

1) Vg. Carlson, K.E.: The Use of Gravity in Isometric Exercises, Am. Exercises—Clinical Usage, J. Nat. Athletic

Coplin, Thomas H.: Isokinetic Exercises—Clinical Usage, J. Nat. Athletic Trainers Ass. 6 (1971) 3, p. 110.

Hettinger, Theodor: Isometrisches Muskeltraining, Stuttgart 1972

Hinson, M.; J. Rosentsweig: Comparing the Three Best Ways of Developing Strength, Scholastic Coach 4 (March 1972), p. 34.

Kruger, Arnd: Isokinetisches Krafttraining, Leistungssport 1 (1971) 1, pp. 22-31.

2) Vgl. Oberdieck, Helmut; Arnd Kruger: Die Einordnung physiotherapeutischer Massnahmen in den Trainingsprozess; Leistungsport 1 (1971) pp. 19-30.

FURTHER LITERATURE

Abrahams, Adolphe: The Disabilities and Injuries of Sport, London 1961.

Battista, E.; P. Dumas; F. Macorigh: Soins du Sportif, Paris 1969.

Bould, C.: Hints on Athletic Injuries (Amateur Athletic Assn.) London (1960).

Firth, D.: Cold as an Adjunctive Modality: J. Am. Osteopathic Assn. 70 (March 1971), p. 715-716.

Heiss, Frohwalt: Unfallverhutung beim Sport, Schorndorf 1972.

Mayhew, J.L.: Effects of Ankle Taping on Motor Performance, J. Nat. Athletic Trainers Assn. 7 (March 1972), p. 10-11.

Muckle, David S.: Sports Injuries, Newcastle upon Tyne 1971.

Nocker, Josef: Physiologie der Leibesubungen, Stuttgart 1971.

Schultz, Erich; Karl E. Rothschuh: Bau und Funktionen des menschlichen Korpers, Munchen 1971.

The American College of Sports Medicine (Ed.): Encyclopedia of Sport Sciences and Medicine, New York 1971.

Thomas, J.R.; D.J. Cotten: Does Ankle Taping Slow Down Athletes? Coach and Athlete 34 (Nov. 1971), p. 20.

Wood, J.P.: The Traumatized Knee Joint, A Statistical Review, J. Am. Osteopathic Assn. 70 (April 1971), p. 776-782.

Host, Charles P. (Ed.): Sports Safety—Accident Prevention and Injury Control in Physical Education, Athletics and Recreation, Washington, D.C. (1971).

Allman, Fred L.: What a Trainer Ought to be: Journal of National American Trainers Association (Nata), 5 (1970), 3, pp. 3-7.

Bryant, Jim: Contributions of Athletic Trainers to Human Dignity: Journal of Nata, 5 (1970), 3, pp. 13-14.

Cha, Donald A.; Gerald Smith: Controlled Speed and Accommodating Resistance, Journal of Nata, 6 (1971) 1.

Hoffa/Gocht/Storck: Technik der Massage, Stuttgart 1949.

Klafs, Carl E.; Daniel D. Arnheim: Modern Principles of Athletic Training, St. Louis, Mo. 1969.

Kraus, J.F.; et al.: Injury Reporting and Recording: Some Essential Elements in the Collection and Retrieval of Sports-Injury Information, J. of Am. Med. Assn., 213 (1970) July 20, p. 438-447.

Leuthard, F.: Lehrbuch der Physiologischen Chemie, Berlin 1963.

Marshall, W.: The Psychology of Being Hurt, J. of Louisiana Med. Soc., 122

(1970) June, p. 180-184.

Oberdieck, Helmut: Die VII. Europameisterschaften der Leichtathletik 1962 im Spiegel der Sportsmassagebetreuung, Zeitschrift der deutschen, Badebetrieb 1963/64, Lubeck.

O'Donoghue, D.H.: Treatment of Injuries of Athletes, Philadelphia 1962.

Rohrbach, Wilhelm: Lehrbuch der Bader- und Massagekunde, Lubeck 1960.

Sayers; Miller: Approval of Athletic Training Curriculum at Colleges and Universities, Journal of Nata, 5 (1970) 2, p. 10f.

Sullivan, George F.: Conditioning Procedures in Prevention of Knee Injuries, Journal of Nata, 4 (1969) 2, p. 12 f.

Thorndike, A.: Athletic Injuries, Philadelphia 1962.

STRETCHING

CHART FOR RUNNERS

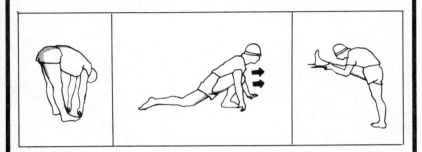

A jumbo 22½ x 34" wall chart, prepared by stretching expert Bob Anderson. 17 "before running" stretches, fully illustrated and described (whole series takes 10 min.), plus 14 "after running" stretches (12 min.), all designed to keep you injury-free and on the run. The importance of proper stretching to running fitness cannot be over-emphasized, and this large-sized wall chart enables you to easily incorporate regular stretching into your routine. Stretches for the Achilles, hamstrings, quadriceps, back and stomach muscles, groin, calf, thigh, etc.

STRETCHING CHART FOR RUNNERS is available from Track & Field News, Box 296, Los Altos, CA 94022 for $2.50, postage paid. Calif. residents add 12¢ sales tax.

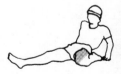